248.4
BRA

17964

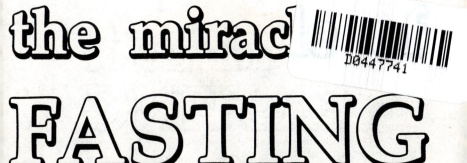

the mirac̶l̶e̶

FASTING

PROVEN THROUGHOUT HISTORY
For Physical, Mental and Spiritual Rejuvenation

Learn to Live in Agelessness With
BRAGG'S COMPLETE
LIFE EXTENSION PROGRAM

PAUL C. BRAGG, N.D., Ph.D.
LIFE EXTENSION SPECIALIST
and
PATRICIA BRAGG, N.D., Ph.D.
LIFE EXTENSION NUTRITIONIST

The Bragg Crusades for a 100% Healthy, Better World for All!

Library
HEALTH SCIENCE   Oakland S.U.M.

Box 7, Santa Barbara, California 93102 U.S.A

the miracle of
FASTING

By
PAUL C. BRAGG, N.D., Ph.D.
LIFE EXTENSION SPECIALIST

Copyright © 1985 by Health Science. All rights reserved under the International Copyright Union. Printed in the United States of America. No portion of this book may be reproduced or used in any manner without the written permission of the publisher, except by a reviewer who wishes to use brief quotations in a review for a magazine, newspaper, or radio or television program. For information address Health Science, Box 7, Santa Barbara, California, 93102, USA.

Thirty-Fourth Printing MCMLXXXV

Revised 1985

Library of Congress Catalog Card No. 84-062771

ISBN: 0-87790-035-3

Health Science - Box 7, Santa Barbara, CA. 93102

Health   Peace
Happiness   Youthfulness
Love   Joy
Praise   Patience
Vitality   Fortitude
Strength   Charity
        Faith

I Dedicate this Book to Eight Men of Great Wisdom — men
whom I owe my Health and my Long Vigorous, Happy Life.

Dr. August Rollier, M.D. —
    Father of Heliotheraphy (Sunshine Theraphy).
Bernarr Macfadden —
    Father and Founder of the Physical
    Culture Movement
Prof. Arnold Ehret —
    Originator of the Mucusless Diet Healing
    System.
Dr. St. Louis Estes, D.D.S. —
    One of the greatest and most dynamic
    speakers for Natural Nutrition.
Dr. Benedict Lust, M.D. —
    Father and Founder of Naturopathy in America.
Dr. John Harvey Kellogg, M.D. —
    For 60 years the Director of the Famous
    Battle Creek Sanitarium in Battle Creek,
    Michigan.
Dr. Henry Lindlahr, M.D. —
    Famous Drugless Physician, who pioneered for
    the return to Natural Method of treatment.
Dr. John T. Tilden, M.D. —
    Great Natural Healer

Paul C. Bragg

Patricia Bragg

BRAGG BLESSINGS FROM OUR HOME

From the Bragg home to your home we share our years of health knowledge—years of living close to God and Nature and what joys of fruitful, radiant living this produces—this my Father and I share with you and your loved ones.

With Blessings for Health and Happiness,

Patricia Bragg

Foreword

MEDICAL SCIENCE REDISCOVERS FASTING
WITH REMARKABLE RESULTS

..As the last quarter of the 20th century approaches, medical science in both the USA and the USSR is rediscovering Nature's original healing method...Fasting...with results often hailed as "sensational".

Called the "hunger cure" in Russia, distilled water fasts up to 45 days have been reported by Soviet doctors as successful treatment for a wide variety of disorders...including those of the skin and metabolism, bronchial asthma, hypertension, gallstones, tumors, pancreatitis, early forms of artery hardening, and arthritis.

The most spectacular results of "controlled hunger" treatment were reported in 1972 by Dr. Yuri Nikolayev of the Moscow Research Institute of Psychiatry, where some 7,000 patients with psychic disorders, primarily sluggish forms of schizophrenia, have responded positively to fasting.

Stressing that such treatment should be undertaken only under carefully controlled conditions, Dr. Nikolayev said, "The hunger treatment gives the entire nervous system and the brain a rest. The body is cleaned of poisons and the tissues and glands renovated. Resting the brain forms the basis for the treatment of neuropsychic disorders."

Fasting is also being used in psychiatric treatment in the United States. Seriously ill schzophrenics were treated in a hospital on distilled water fasts of 16 to 81 days by a Northern California psychiatrist, according to a 1972 report.

Fasting is also being used in the treatment of various disorders at the Philadelphia General Hospital. Veterans Hospitals and other leading medical institutions throughout the country. Watch for reports on the results.

Paul C. Bragg, who has supervised fasts for many thousands of people during the past 60-odd years...with results that are frequently termed "miraculous"...finds it "encouraging and gratifying that medical science is at last rediscovering the treatment prescribed by the father of medicine, Hippocrates...Nature's own prescription...the Miracle of Fasting!"

Our Favorite Quotes We Share With You
(you will find them where space allows)

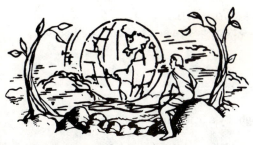

CONTENTS

"To preserve health is a moral and religious duty, for health is the basis for all social virtues. We can no longer be useful when not well."
— Dr. Samuel Johnson, Father of Dictionaries

◇◇

Contents

◇◇

Chapters

Fasting clears away the thousand little things which quickly accumulate and clutter the heart and mind. It cuts through the corrosion, renewing our contact with God.

They ministered to the Lord, and fasted.

--Acts 13:2 R.V.

GETTING THE MOST OUT OF LIFE

Every thinking person, must at one time or the other say to himself, "Am I getting the most out of life"?

I credit the great comedian, Ed Wynn, with making a profound remark, he said, "Without health, riches, possessions, and fame are all mud."

What is man without health, even though endowed with riches and fame? Riches cannot buy happiness. Because a person has achieved fame it does not follow that he is happy.

I do not discredit riches. I think money and possessions have their place in our culture. Physical comforts and luxuries are most important to many people. Take away a man's wealth and give him only health and his first desire will be the return of his riches.

But with both achieved a word remains which we hate to utter; a thought we dread to contemplate; a thing which gives sorrow, pain and grief. That word, that thought, that thing, is DEATH. Even in cases where life appears a burden, how tenaciously does man cling to it! How the spirit recoils from a struggle with DEATH! How fondly it retains its grasp on life! Man's great desire is for health and long life on earth; "Man clings to the world as his home, and would want to live here forever, if he had health and long-lasting youthfulness."

I LOVE LIFE AND I WANT TO LIVE!

At my health lectures I often sing my favorite song for my students called, "I Love Life, and I Want to Live". These strong words express the inner desires of each one of us. Life in itself is a miracle. And you and I who have life are holding this miracle in the palms of our hands.

Life is Precious...It is the Treasure of Treasures

Since Adam and Eve lived in that historic Garden of Eden, the prolongation of human life has been the most fascinating problem that has challenged the attention of mankind. The Persian and Greek sages, centuries before Christ summoned their intellectual forces to solve it, but in vain.

The scholasticism of the Medieval Ages took it up zealously, but with kindred results, and today, in this twentieth century, every intelligent mind seeks, though often blindly, its solution.

No man since the dawn of creation has escaped Death; yet each individual, by harkening to Hygienic and Dietetic truth, and barring accident, can live to an advanced age. Every person owes it to himself, his relatives, his friends and to his country, to care for his body, that its healthy action may make him a valued citizen, that the years of his life may be extended to their normal limit. I believe every person is entitled to his 120 years or more of life as the Bible states.

Longevity may be defined as the duration of life that a healthy person attains, under the most favorable conditions.

DAILY LIVING HABITS KILLING AMERICANS!

Man by his imprudence in diet, drink, and manifold excesses, dies before one-half of his potential life has been lived.

Wild animals, undisturbed, live out their full term of life. Man is the only exception. Of human kind, not more than one in a million lives out his natural limit. Animals in their wild, untrammeled state know by instinct how to live, and what to eat and drink. They fast when they get hurt or sick.

By instinct, animals are led to eat what is wholesome for them, but man eats and drinks anything and everything - consuming the most indigestible concoctions, washes it down with poisonous slops, and then wonders why he does not live to be a centenarian!

In theory, we all desire long life - in practice, we abbreviate our lives to the minimum. Does this make sense?

Why this marvelous mechanism of man - perfect in its minutest organism, combining a God-like intelligence with a body which sculptors have imitated but never equalled - should be ruthlessly destroyed by himself, is one of the inexplicable wonders of our creation!

The marble statue of Apollo which the writer saw in the Vatican at Rome, a world famous work of art, is not greater in the perfection of manly beauty than that possessed by thousands of young men in our midst today; yet the inanimate marble Apollo is as tenderly cared for as a priceless jewel, while the living man, noble, intellectual and refined, with a delicate and sensitive physical structure, gives this wonderful body of his less attention than he gives to his cat or dog.

All people of sound mentality, desire a long, happy, useful life. With our intelligence, longevity and super-health should be the rule, but alas, it is the exception.

SICKNESS IS A CRIME - DON'T BE A CRIMINAL

At the turn of the century I was associated with the great Bernarr Macfadden, Father and Founder of the Physical Culture movement. I was associate Editor of the magazine Physical Culture. The front cover of that magazine always carried these lines "SICKNESS IS A CRIME - DON'T BE A CRIMINAL".

Physical weakness, flabbiness and sickness have always seemed criminal to me as well as sacrilegious abuse of that wonderful instrument, the human body. Ever since I regained my health from a hopeless, helpless cripple many years ago, I've made a religion of keeping in perfect health by conscientious care of my body. Adhering to a high ideal of stamina, vitality, health and endurance it has paid me dividends - such priceless, dividends that I call myself "A Health Billionaire".

To be A Health Billionaire... To Enjoy the Glow
Of Ageless Health - You Must Work For It.

The "secret" of the glow of ageless health lies in internal cleanliness and regeneration through natural, organically grown live foods and other regenerative principles such as fasting, pure air, exercise, relaxation, etc.

When you purify your body with systematic fasting and live foods you crave daily exercise. And by exercise you sculpture your body to become the person you want to be.

Just think, from this minute on... YOU... will mold your body to physical perfection.

With the knowledge found in these pages you will find out how YOU... can get the most out of life!

Man is a unique study to say the least, a very intriguing one, but the laws which govern man's being are quite simple and very understandable if one takes the time to learn and to observe how he functions from day to day.

LIFE CAN BE A HAPPY AND JOYOUS ADVENTURE

To know one's self seems like an endless task, but with crystal clear observation and the daily application of these simple but precise laws, life becomes not only a most exciting adventure, but a tremendous joy. It behooves every one of us to embark upon this Health Course of Life. Study and continue it throughout the years, and really experience day by day the joys, happiness and pleasures of a healthy, happy, long and vigorous life.

Paul C. Bragg

Life Extension Specialist

I humbled my soul with fasting.

--Psalm 69:10

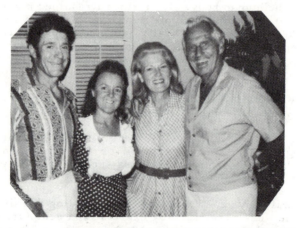

Jack LaLanne, Patricia Bragg, Elaine LaLanne & Paul Bragg

Jack says, "Bragg saved my life at age 14 when I attended the Bragg Health & Fitness Lecture in Oakland, California." From that day on, Jack has lived the health life and teaches Health & Fitness to millions every morning with his T.V. Exercise Show.

THE MIRACLE OF FASTING

2

What, in your opinion, is the most significant discovery of this modern age?

The finding of Dinosaur eggs on the plains of Mongolia, which scientists assert were laid some 10,000,000 years ago?

The unearthing of ancient tombs and cities, with their confirmation of the Scriptural story, and their matchless specimens of bygone civilization?

The radioactive time clock by which Professor Lane of Tufts College estimates the age of the earth of 1,250,000,000 years?

Jet airplanes? Television? Radio? Atomic Energy? The Hydrogen Bomb?

NO — NOT ANY OF THESE!

THE GREATEST DISCOVERY OF MODERN TIMES

In my opinion, the greatest discovery by modern man is the power to rejuvenate himself physically, mentally, and spiritually with RATIONAL FASTING.

With scientific fasting, man can create within himself a quality of agelessness.

With fasting, man may check premature aging.

The dread of "Growing Old" and becoming a burden to himself and others is one of man's greatest fears.

The fear of being senile, helpless, and unable to care for one's self is deep in every thinking person's heart.

With the complete knowledge of Fasting as outlined in this course of instruction ... you can banish all your fears of premature aging. With a 24-hour complete water-fast weekly, making 52 days a year of body purification and at least three 7- to 10-day fasts yearly ... you can keep the rust and cinders from your movable joints and muscles. You must bear in mind it is the debris of metabolism (biological process of converting food into living matter, and the matter into energy) that brings on many of your physical miseries and premature aging.

When the "Vital Force" of your Body drops below normal, then all your physical problems as well as your mental ones begin.

FASTING CONSERVES YOUR "VITAL FORCE"

Let me explain ... We eat food and, as it passes through the body, it must be masticated, digested, assimilated and then the waste is eliminated. We have four great organs of elimination ... the bowels, the kidneys, the lungs, and the skin.

In order for these eliminative organs to work perfectly, the body must build a high "Vital Force" or energy quota.

It Takes Energy To Eliminate Body Wastes

It takes a tremendous amount of "Vital Energy" to pass a large meal through the gastro-intestinal tract ... the thirty-foot tube that runs from the mouth to the rectum.

It takes the great power of "Vital Energy" to pass liquids through the 2 million filters of the human kidneys. It takes "Vital Power" for the chemical power of the liver and the gall bladder to do their work in preparing food for the billions of body cells to feed upon.

It takes great "Vital Power" for the lungs to bring in oxygen to purify the whole 5 to 8 quarts of blood in your body, and expel carbon dioxide.

It takes great "Vital Power" for the skin, with its 96 million pores, to throw off body poisons in the form of moisture and sweat.

✸ ✸ ✸ ✸ ✸

To lengthen thy life, Lessen they meals.

✸

Who is strong? He that can conquer his bad habits.
　　　　　　　　　　　　　　　　　　　　　 – Ben Franklin

WE LIVE IN A POISONED WORLD

It is the duty of the "Vital Power" to supply the energy to rid the body of the poisons that are created in our intake of food. The "Vital Power" must keep the body temperature at 98.6 degrees at all times --- if it goes higher, we become sick --- if we fall below this figure, we become sick.

In our modern civilization, the "Vital Power" has many other poisons to cope with — the filth and dirt that man creates.

THE BIG FILTHY SEWER IN THE SKY ABOVE US

We are bombarded with noxious and harmful, filthy, dirt from our skies. Take New York City as an example ... roughly 60 tons of airborne dust particles fall on each square mile every month.

Think of the sky dirt the body must battle with to keep a person in New York alive. No wonder there are so many hospitals and sick people in that poisoned city.

Scientists estimate that an inhabitant of an industrial city such as Pittsburgh or Birmingham, Ala., stands a better than average chance of contracting a deadly lung disease or suffering from heart trouble, just by breathing polluted air. That special form of poisoned air known as smog regularly affects not only Los Angeles, but Phoenix, Chicago, St. Louis, Kansas City, Washington, and many other cities and towns across the nation.

A grim mixture of soot and smoke from factories, incinerators, and heating plants; the gaseous by-products of industry; and the exhaust fumes of cars and trucks are making an ugly mess out of most of the air Americans breathe. Air pollution is a real menace to our health and life. And fasting is our only salvation in helping to get these filthy poisons out of our body!

Further on in this book, I will explain how to examine your urine. After a few days of fasting, you will actually be able to see some of the poisons your body contained.

OUR RIVERS, LAKES, STREAMS, AND CREEKS ARE FILLED WITH POLLUTION

Not only does air fill our body with poisons, but our water is so filthy that powerful chemicals are used to make it fit to drink.

An inorganic mineral called chlorine is used to help purify our drinking water ... as well as alum and many other inorganic minerals. Remember, your body can only absorb organic minerals (from the vegetable and animal kingdom). Any inorganic mineral must be eliminated from the body by the "Vital Power".

If the "Vital Power" is below normal, then many of these inorganic chemicals are stored in the body tissues to cause future trouble. Lake Erie is critically ill, and the symptoms are there for all to see. Beaches that once were gleaming with white sand are covered with odorous green slime. The lake's prize fish, walleyes, blue pike, yellow perch, and whitefish have all but disappeared, and the fishing has fled along with them. One Cleveland health student wrote me "Our lake is a wastebasket for factories. It is unfit for fish to live in, and for people to drink, because it is loaded with deadly chemicals". The major reason for the lake's terrible pollution is that most of its larger tributaries have turned into little more than open sewers. Detroit alone pours 1.5 million gallons of waste a day into the Detroit River, which flows directly into Lake Erie.

The Cuyahoga River, which runs through the middle of Akron and Cleveland, before spilling into the lake, is so clogged with logs, rotted pilings, flammable chemicals, oil slicks, and old tires, that it has been labeled the filthiest water in America. Added to the scum and stench are thousands of dead fish that were smothered by the nasty pollution.

On a cruise up the Buffalo River last summer, Buffalo's mayor slid past islands of detergents, pools of grain dust, and a general rainbow of dirty industrial discharge. The stink was overpowering. "Unbelievable! Disgusting!" he concluded.

I am citing only one water supply among the many that are completely contaminated. All across this great country of ours we find our water supply polluted. We must use water ... lots of it, and all of it must be heavily chemicalized to be fit to use.

And REMEMBER ... all those inorganic chemicals must be passed out of your body or they can cause great damage.

If the "Vital Power" of the body drops and cannot force these inorganic chemicals through our eliminative systems ... then they remain in our bodies and cause great trouble and damage.

If we are to get these poisons out of our body --- we must Fast --- by Fasting we give our body a physiological rest --- this rest builds our "Vital Power" and the more "Vital Power" we have, the more poisons and toxins are going to be eliminated from our bodies.

Fasting Is For Internal Cleansing And Purification.

8

POISONING FROM CHEMICAL SPRAYS

Tons upon tons of all kinds of deadly sprays are not only sprayed in the air to kill insects, but many more tons are sprayed on our sick fruits and vegetables.

Salads are healthy and appetizing, but often are deadly because of the use of insecticide sprays.

This year's crop of fruit and vegetables are exposed to more poisonous pesticide chemicals than ever before. You should constantly be on guard to protect your health.

Beware of that salad --- it may fill your body with deadly poisons. A group of women were having lunch at a Miami hotel, and shortly afterwards, they were all seized with an attack of cramps. Then, nausea and dizziness followed. Pale and shaken from vomiting, the women were prostrate, until medical aid arrived.

It didn't take the physician long to trace the source of this outbreak of acute poisoning. The villain was an appetizing green salad, consisting of lettuce, tomatoes, and a touch of dressing. In giving his reasons for the illness, the doctor said: The poisoning was caused by an overdose of DDT, and other sprays on the salad vegetables."

CROPS EXPOSED TO POISON

More and more poisonous pesticide chemicals are being put on our food. As early as March, the Food and Drug Administration announced: "Three seizures were made of salad vegetables contaminated with excess residues of pesticide chemicals. Two shipments of endive were charged to exceed the legal tolerance of parathion (one of the most deadly poisons in use). A shipment of lettuce was seized because of high residues of DDT."

Three shipments were seized, but this doesn't tell the whole sad story of food poisoning. First of all, only shipments destined for interstate commerce are checked, and only a small fraction of the total produce ever comes under the scrutiny of an inspector. Many tons and truckloads of lettuce containing pesticide residues "in excess of legal tolerance" will stay within the state or community where grown. They will not be checked at all. And as far as shipments across state lines are concerned, the Food and Drug Administration will be first to admit that, because of limited manpower, only a tiny fraction of the vegetable shipments in interstate commerce are checked.

★ ★ ★ ★ ★

Some students drink deeply at the fountain of knowledge - others only gargle.

The frightening truth is that a high percentage of the field crops reaching your salad bowl and your vegetable juicer have been sprayed with a wide variety of deadly poisons; among them, chlorinated hydrocarbons including DDT, phosphorous compounds, and a number of weed killers. The contamination of salad vegetables doesn't stop with spraying the leafy portion of the plant. Medical researchers have discovered that DDT and other agricultural chemicals, such as fertilizers, applied to the soil remain there for many months, and are picked up constantly by succeeding crops grown in the fields. The poison finally ends up in the pulp of the vegetable itself. It is part of it and cannot be washed off. I suppose it has occurred to you that, if the vegetables in your salad are contaminated, you should make some effort to get rid of the residue before you eat too much of it. You might feel that peeling the skin of a tomato or removing the outer layer of the lettuce will do the job. It won't. Some of the residue will be removed, certainly, but there will be more in lower leaves, and in the pulp. The chemicals cannot even be broken down by cooking. The poison is there to stay.

FASTING AIDS IN FLUSHING DEADLY POISONS FROM THE BODY

When we fast --- stop eating --- all the "Vital Power" that has been used to convert food into energy and body tissue, is now used to flush poisons from the body!

In my own personal life, for instance, I travel all over the United States and the entire world, lecturing. I am fortunate knowing health-minded people throughout the world — so am usually well-supplied with homegrown, organically grown fruits and vegetables from their small gardens. But I am often forced to eat the food I find wherever I am. I know most of it has been sprayed with deadly poisons ... that is the reason I fast one complete 24- to 36-hour period of each week, as well as doing four 10-day fasting periods per year.

When I go on a 10-day complete water-fast, each day I take a specimen of my urine the first thing upon arising ... I put it in a small bottle and let it cool and settle. In a few days I can see little crystals forming in the urine ... I have had my urine examined for chemicals, and the examiner has told me time and time again that traces of DDT, and other deadly pesticide residues, appeared in my urine.

On one occasion I took a 21-day complete fast --- on the 19th day I had terrible pains in my bladder --- when I urinated it felt like red hot water passing through me. I had the urine examined and sure enough it was filled with DDT and other deadly pesticide poisons.

10

A great feeling of energy flowed over my body when this poison passed out of my body. The whites of my eyes were as clear as new snow --- my body took on a pink glow --- and energy surged through my body. Now, remember I had been fasting for 19 days --- yet I drove over to Pasadena, California, to Mt. Wilson, which is six thousand feet high, and climbed the trail with absolutely no exertion. I ran most of the way down the winding trail. I felt that a tremendous burden had been lifted from my body. In my personal opinion, fasting is the only way to rid the body of commercial poisons found in our fruits and vegetables.

APPETIZING FRUITS AND VEGETABLES ARE OFTEN COATED WITH A WAX THAT CAN BE A MENACE TO YOUR HEALTH

Top medical experts reveal the newest menace to the Nation's health. Next time you eat an apple, pear, plum, green pepper, or cucumber, take a good look at its surface. Is it bright and shiny? Does it have a smooth, glossy look? If it has ... BEWARE!

Chances are that it has been coated with a wax paraffin solution which according to eminent medical experts ... presents one of America's most serious health threats. The wax coating seals fruits and vegetables with a protective layer which retains the water and juices ... preserving the taste and appearance of freshness. But it may also leave residues that can harm your body.

What you are eating, therefore, is a kind of wax that cannot be handled by your body — a paraffin wax, a by-product of petroleum. There is no organ in your body, including the liver, that can handle petroleum. This deadly wax therefore runs wild in the body. That is the reason doctors are so baffled by the many new diseases that American people are acquiring from foods that are being contaminated by commercial interests.

We must not let this wax remain in our bodies to cause damage. Therefore, in my opinion, I believe the weekly 24- to 36-hour fast and the longer fasts during the year will aid in ridding our bodies of this deadly petroleum wax.

Keep this constantly in mind when you are on a complete fast ... there is a large amount of "Vital Power" to do the needed clean-up work in the body!

✷ ✷ ✷ ✷ ✷

"Medicine is only palliative", says Dr. Weir Mitchell "For back of disease lies the cause, and this cause no drug can reach."

POWERFUL NEW POISONS INVADE YOUR DIET

Many of the 1,000 or more synthetic food additives dumped into the nation's food supply are responsible for a great deal of sickness. For many years, our foods have been loaded with so-called "safe" chemicals that have now been discovered to be harmful to the human body ... and many of them are still being used!

Take a loaf of commercially refined white bread ... this bread has been treated, bleached, colored, dyed, enriched, purified, softened, preserved, flavored, and given a fresh odor ... all by synthetic chemicals.

It is almost impossible to get a loaf of 100% whole grain bread that is free of sprays and synthetic food additives.

The human body is a collection of individual cells, nothing more. If nourished by a food supply which provides basic needs for growth and normal function to sustain life, those cells may go on for as long as 120 years or more! But when man toys with his environment and pollutes it with foul, dirty air, naturally certain of his cells may respond adversely and he is sent to his sick bed or to the graveyard. When he pollutes his food, and changes its entire composition with synthetic chemicals, it follows that other body cells may be damaged, function poorly, and be unable to adjust to the irritating substances supplied.

How can the body function in top physical condition
when it is loaded with synthetic food additives?

My only answer is to eat foods that are as close to natural as possible ... keep away from the complicated, chemicalized, preserved foods. Eat as many organically-grown foods as you can possibly obtain. Read the labels of all foods you purchase! Ask questions about any special food you like ... even write the company which produces the food and ask for a complete analysis.

Fast 24- to 36-hours weekly to get rid of as much commercial dirt as possible. When you do not feel up to par ... take a 7 to 10-day complete fast and give your body a thorough house-cleaning. You will be amazed how much of this commercial poison has crept into your food. Remember the commercial interests are not interested in your health and life ... they are only looking for your hard-earned cash.

★ ★ ★ ★ ★

Dine with little, sup with less; do better still:
sleep supperless.   Ben Franklin

When you fast ... the "Vital Power" is doing a cleansing job for you.

- The body is self-cleansing, self-healing, and self-repairing!

- When you stop eating, wonderful things happen in your body!

- If we are going to keep our bodies clean --- we must fast!

- Just try fasting a few times --- you will get a feeling you have never had before --- internal cleaning will put you on the road to Health.

SALT - WHAT YOU DON'T KNOW ABOUT THIS COMMON PRODUCT WILL STARTLE YOU!

Would you use sodium, a caustic alkali, to season your food? Or chlorine, a poisonous gas? "Ridiculous questions," you say. "Nobody would be foolhardy enough to do that."

Of course not. But the shocking truth is that most people do so ... because they don't know that these powerful chemicals constitute the inorganic crystaline compound known as SALT.

For centuries, the expression "salt of the earth" has been used as a catch-all phrase to designate something good and essential. Nothing could be more erroneous. For that harmless product that you shake into your food every day may actually bury you. Consider these startling facts:

1. SALT IS NOT A FOOD! There is no more justification for its culinary use than there is for potassium chloride, calcium chloride, barium chloride, or any other chemical on the druggist's shelf.

2. Salt cannot be digested, assimilated, or utilized by the body. Salt has no nutritional value! SALT HAS NO VITAMINS! NO ORGANIC MINERALS! NO NUTRIENTS OF ANY KIND! Instead, it is positively harmful and may bring on troubles in the kidneys, bladder, heart, arteries, veins, and blood vessels. Salt may waterlog the tissues, causing a dropsical condition.

3. Salt may act as a heart poison. It also increases the irritability of the nervous system.

4. Salt acts to rob calcium from the body and attacks the mucous lining throughout the entire gastrointestional tract. If salt is so dangerous to health, why is it used so widely? Mainly because it is a habit that has become ingrained over thousands of years. But it is a habit based on a serious misconception. The misconception is that the body needs it. But many people, such as the Eskimos, never eat salt, and never miss it. Once a person is free of the habit, salt is as objectionable and repulsive to the taste as tobacco is to a nonsmoker. Among certain animal species, salt acts as a positive poison, particularly in the case of fowl. And swine have been known to die after large doses of it.

HOW DID THE SALT HABIT ORIGINATE

The biochemist, Bunge, explains that in prehistoric times there was a proper balance of sodium and potassium minerals in the earth. But continued rainfall over the centuries washed away the more soluble sodium salts. In time, all soils and land-grown foods became deficient in sodium but high in potassium. The result was that animals and human beings developed a craving for something to replace this deficiency. They found a poor, ineffective, and highly dangerous substitute in inorganic sodium chloride, or common salt.

Swallowing salt to obtain natural sodium is like taking inorganic calcium to get calcium. Both are chemicals, and neither can be assimilated by body cells. Since all inorganic chemicals are harmful to digestive organs, we can understand why the stomach develops a sudden and abnormal thirst after salt is consumed! The stomach is simply reacting to a foreign substance and is taking quick action to wash it out of the body through the kidneys. You can imagine what effect this has on the delicate kidney filters. Of all the body organs, the kidneys are most subject to injury from salt. What happens when more salt is eaten than the kidneys can eliminate? The excess is deposited in various parts of the body, especially in the feet and lower part of the legs. Salt tends to swell the feet and legs.

To protect its tissues against this poison — salt, the body automatically seeks to dilute it by accumulating water in these areas. As the tissues become waterlogged, the body tends to swell. Feet and ankles bloat painfully. Just as salt is harmful to the kidneys, so it is injurious to the heart. Even a small amount of salt is considered, in some heart conditions, to be dangerous! The action of the heart muscle is governed by the relative concentration and balance of natural, organic sodium and calcium salts in the blood, so that an excess of sodium will therefore tend to disturb this action, increasing the heartbeat and the blood pressure.

The Japanese, according to medical statistics, suffer from the highest blood pressure in the world, and they are also known to be the world's highest salt consumers.

WHAT SALT DOES TO YOUR BLOOD PRESSURE

What causes high blood pressure? Medical science knows of many causes: tension, strains, stress, toxic substances such as cigarettes and gasoline fumes, food additives, insecticide sprays, the side effects of drugs, and industrialization are suspect. What can you do to protect yourself from these causative agents? It is well to exclude as many of these harmful agents from your environment as possible!

However, there is one cause of high blood pressure which can be remedied. Sodium chloride (common table salt) is the major cause of high blood pressure.

Up to now, we have been talking about causing high blood pressure in the "normal" person. But how about the effects of salt on those millions suffering from our country's most prevalent ailment, OVERWEIGHT. Here is a sensitive area for research, because overweight is known to be frequently accompanied by high blood pressure. Is there a link between the overweight individual's high blood pressure and his salt intake?

THE MYTH OF THE "SALT LICK"

Is a low-salt diet a deficient diet? Don't we need plenty of salt in our diets to keep us in top physical condition? This is a popular notion ... but is it true? People will tell you that animals will travel for miles to visit the so-called "salt licks". I investigated the salt-licks where wild forest animals congregated from miles around to lick the soil. Although all of these sites were known as "salt licks" the one chemical property they all had in common was complete absence of sodium chloride (common salt). There was absolutely NO organic or inorganic sodium at the salt licks. But they had an abundance of many organic minerals and nutrients which the animals craved.

WHY COWS ARE GIVEN LARGE AMOUNTS OF SALT

A man who puts his investment in a dairy farm is in it to make all the profit he can. Therefore dairy men have found that by giving cows salt blocks to lick, they will drink more water ... the more water they drink, the more milk the cow will produce. But the result is that a quart of milk contains the extremely high content of 1-1/2 grams of salt per quart. For a five-month old infant, this is equivalent to 1/2 ounce of salt to an adult. Go past any American school and look at the bodies of the different children ... you will be amazed how many of them are obese, being many pounds overweight. They are heavy drinkers of commercial milk, and most of their food has high concentrations of salt. Go into your supermarkets across the country and look at the canned and bottled foods ... all of them are loaded with salt. Salt in the milk ... salt in the vegetables and other foods. Add it up and you can see why heart disease is the number one killer in our country. We are a nation of salt drunkards! Cheese, canned vegetables, bread, in fact all our most popular foods are saturated with salt. Baby foods are loaded with SALT!

WE ARE TOLD WE MUST TAKE SALT TABLETS IN HOT WEATHER

Most people have the preconceived idea that salt lost in perspiring must be immediately replaced. In many factories, the management supplies salt tablets to keep the workers in "good health" but, are these salt tablets necessary? In my opinion "NO"!

MY HIKE ACROSS DEATH VALLEY, CALIFORNIA - THE HOTTEST SPOT IN THE WORLD

To prove definitely to myself that I did not need salt during extremely hot weather, I went to Death Valley, California, one of the hottest spots in the entire world during July and August. On my first test I hired 10 husky young college athletes to make the hike from Furnace Creek Ranch in Death Valley to Stovepipe Wells, a distance of approximately 30 miles. I gave the college athletes all the salt tablets and all the water they could drink ... and a station wagon carried plenty of food that contained salt foods, bread, buns, crackers, cheese, lunch meats, hot dogs, thus allowing them to eat, drink, and take salt tablets as they desired. I had no salt ... and, on that 30-mile hike, I fasted. The hike was started at the end of July ... the thermometer stood at 105 degrees. We started the hike a little after eight in the morning --- the higher the sun rose, the more cruel the blazing hot sun became, up and up went the thermometer until at 12 noon it stood at 130 degrees ... a dry hot heat, that seemed to want to melt you!

The college boys gobbled the salt tables and guzzled quarts of cool water ... at lunch they ate ham sandwichs, drank cola drinks, and cheese sandwiches. We rested a half-hour after lunch and continued our rugged hike across the red-hot blazing sands. Soon things were beginning to happen to the strong, husky college boys ... first, three of them got violently ill and threw up all they ate and drank for lunch ... they got dizzy and turned deathly pale and a great weakness overcame them. They quit the hike cold! They were driven back to the Furnace Creek Ranch in poor condition. But the hike went on with seven college athletes continuing. As we hiked, they drank large amounts of water and took salt tablets. Then suddenly five of them got stomach cramps and became deathly ill. Up came the water and some of the lunch --- these five had to be driven back to the ranch.

That left but two out of ten hikers ... it was now about 4 p.m. and the merciless sun beat down on us with great fury ... almost to the second, the last remaining salt-tablet athletes collapsed in the hot burning sun and had to be rushed back to the ranch for medical care.

ONLY NON-SALT USER FINISHES HIKE

That left great-grandfather Bragg alone on the test and I felt as fresh as a daisy! I was not full of salt tablets and I was not full of food because I was on a complete fast. I drank only the warm water I needed ... the college boys wanted cold water, but I drank warm water. I finished the 30-mile hike in around 10-1/2 hours ... and I had no ill effects whatsoever! I camped out for the night and next day arose and hiked another 30 miles back to the ranch without food or salt tablets.

The medical doctors gave me a thorough examination and found me in perfect condition. I am ready and willing to repeat this hike across Death Valley, California, for any scientific group that wants to do research on salt.

MORE PROOF SALT NOT NEEDED

Rommel's German-Afrikan Corps swept across the gates of Egypt, fought, and lost a hard battle before El Alamein, retreating over hundreds of miles of blazing desert; yet, when the campaign was over, the English found captured troops in good physical condition, even though the Nazi soldiers were not supplied with salt tablets.

This story, just as my own, which was performed in the blazing sun of Death Valley, supports the findings of many experiments performed with a non-salt diet on humans under hot desert conditions.

What happens, according to the scientific studies, is this: after the first few days of acclimatization, the subjects cease to lose salt through perspiration. Apparently, there is a normalizing body mechanism at work that conserves the sodium in the body. The comfortable endurance, during all ordinary weather conditions, of people on rigid salt-poor diets shows that this need (for added salt in hot weather) has been greatly exaggerated.

★ ★ ★ ★ ★

Ruts long traveled - grow comfortable.

There is actually enough NATURAL SODIUM in vegetables, fish, meats and other foods, even though they have not been processed with common salt in any way, to supply the needed natural, sodium required by our body. Proof of this fact is found in the known past history of many peoples throughout the world who never used salt.

The American Indians, when the first explorers arrived, knew nothing about the use of salt. Columbus and all of the great explorers of the American continent found wonderful physical specimens when they arrived. The degeneration of the natives always follows the instruction of salt, alcohol, and devitalized foods.

I have made over 13 expeditions to the far primitive corners of the earth and I never found the natives salt users. Therefore none of them suffered with high blood pressure. In fact, regardless of age, they generally had blood pressures of 120 over 80, which is perfect. They suffered from no kidney or heart diseases.

HOW MUCH SALT CAN THE BODY TOLERATE DAILY?

There has been a great deal of research on this subject. The opinion of the research scientists varies from one-half a gram up to one gram of salt per day that can be tolerated by the body. The average American who is a salt addict actually consumes fifteen to thirty times his sodium tolerance each day.

This unfortunately high figure is due to the excessive amount of "hidden salt" in almost all commercially-prepared foods. It is in bread, cheese, prepared meats, (ham, bacon, lunch meats) canned vegetables, and hundreds of other staple foods.

The Southern Negroes have the highest blood pressure in the United States, and data indicates that, for most of them, salt is a prominent item in their diet, salted pork being one of their main staples.

I was born and reared in Virginia and many of my relatives suffered from high blood pressure. They died early of strokes and kidney diseases for they were heavy salt pork eaters, ham eaters, and bacon eaters. High concentrations of salt were used at every meal. By the time these people were 30 years old, they ached all over with what they called the "misery". Their joints were cemented, and they hobbled around stiffly and with pain!

I wonder if the heavy salt diet of the average Southerner brought on this misery? In my opinion, I think so.

★ ★ ★ ★ ★

The best way to lengthen life is to avoid shortening it.

The most dramatic case of salt injury occurred recently in a Binghamton, N. Y., hospital, where a number of babies died when salt was inadvertently used in their formula. An overdose of salt can kill a baby quickly. The body needs natural sodium — organic sodium, not table salt, an inorganic chemical. You can obtain natural sodium which nature provides in ORGANIC FORM ... such as in beets, celery, carrots, potatoes, turnips, sea vegetation, kelp, watercress and many other natural foods. Remember, the organic mineral is the only substance that can be utilized by your living cells.

DE-SALTING BODY CELLS, AND ORGANS BY FASTING

I have had fifty years experience with the science and use of rational fasting. And I have found that in four days of complete fasting we can de-salt the body.

Again the urine will reveal the story of salt to us. Take a four-day complete distilled water fast. Nothing must pass through your body for four complete days, except that you may have all the distilled water you wish to drink!

Each morning take a sample of the first urine the body passes. Put this bottle of urine up on a shelf and let it cool and settle for two or three weeks --- then take it out in the sunlight and look at it ... you will see the concentrated sodium chloride in the bottom of the bottle along with other morbid body wastes. When this salt is passed from the body notice how freely the kidneys will function ... notice how naturally moist your mouth is ... how you have no abnormal thirst. Notice your skin tone, your muscle tone ... there is a thinner and more youthful look to your body. Lumpy waterlogged spots vanish ... the body becomes more streamlined. Bloat is gone and you begin to see your natural figure again. The first thing the body throws off during a fast is salt, and the bloat that goes with it.

You can hardly believe your eyes ... a wonderful transformation is taking place during your fast. The powerful "Vital Force" that would be otherwise used to handle your food is now used exclusively to clean out the debris, the waste, the poisons that have been locked in the body cells and vital organs ... the rejuvenation is taking place in every one of the billions of cells of the body. After the four days of de-salting the body ... keep salt out of the body ... it is a difficult thing to do, as I stated, we find the "hidden salt" in all our foods. That is where your weekly 24- to 36-hour fast helps you de-salt weekly. I often find it difficult, as I travel over the world, lecturing and doing research, to avoid "hidden salt" in foods... even though I always request "No salt, please" in restaurants, on steam ships, airplanes, and trains. However, I feel my weekly fast of 24- to 36-hours keeps

the inorganic salt flowing out of my body. There is never, ever
any salt added to my food. There is no salt ever used in the
Bragg household! We season with herbs and garlic ... which are
the real, natural seasonings. They will put zest in your foods.
With fasting and a low-salt diet, see for yourself how much better
you will feel and look! And what a sweet taste you will always
have in your mouth. You will note many other changes for the
better when you fast and banish the addition of salt from your diet.

FASTING — THE GREAT CLEANSER ... NOT A
CURE FOR ANY HUMAN AILMENT

People are constantly asking and writing me: "Will a fast cure
my 'this or that' disease?" I want it clearly and distinctly understood that I am not recommending FASTING AS A CURE OF
DISEASE! I am not in the curing business. I do not believe in
cures unless nature alone accomplishes the cure. All we can do
is to build up the "Vital Power" of the body so that curing is a
natural internal function of the body alone. I teach you to fast to
build more and more "Vital Power" to overcome enervation and
debilitation.

ENERVATION EXPLAINED

We live in a mad, crazy world. The demands of energy on persons living in this complicated civilization are enormous. We
have a standard living to maintain ... we have a status image to
create before our relations and friends ... Duty is a cruel master
... we must obey our master. Every waking hour is one calling
for great outputs of "Vital Power" to earn our daily living, to
support our family, to drive a car in traffic, to be responsible
for a job, or a house to take care of, rearing children, social
duties, civic duties, the thousands of daily activities that call for
energy and still more energy! Energy is a precious ingredient
--- it cannot be purchased in a bottle or can. Many misguided
persons think they can get it from drugs, alcohol, tobacco, coffee,
tea, and cola drinks, but they are wrong. Energy is a reward for
living as close to natures laws as possible.

We are punished by our bad habits of living and
rewarded by our good habits of living.

It is because of your bad habits of living that things start to
breakdown and decay in your body! Through your bad habits you
enervate or weaken yourself ... and this is the important point
... as your energy drops and you become enervated you do not
have enough energy for your body to cleanse itself properly. Low
energy brings on slow elimination in all the basic eliminative
organs — the bowels, the kidneys, skin and lungs ... no energy

to function at full natural capacity. Then, poisons of all kinds
are not completely flushed out of the body, but lie inside, slowly
building up and taking a terrible toll!

Poisons start to collect in various parts of the body ... they
bring pressure on the nerves of the body, and you suffer from
aches and pains. These are nature's warning signals that you
are not living the way that nature planned the care of your body.
But you blame everything and everybody on your condition,
instead of looking for the real cause.

HUMANS WILL NOT TAKE THE BLAME FOR THEIR MISERIES

"No", they say, "I caught a cold, I worked too hard. I am sick
because I am getting older". Excuse after excuse is given ...
but never the real excuse ... themselves! You and you alone are
responsible for your aches and pains and your premature aging!

By your wrong living you have enervated yourself ... the "Vital
Power" is low ... poisons cannot be flushed out of the body. So,
they find a spot to torment you ... and a name according to the
location of your hurt or pain. But that hurt actually came from
the way you have been living. Do not put the blame elsewhere.
You have lowered or enervated yourself, and the toxic poisons
from many sources of your daily living are tormenting you.
Build the vital energy by fasting and natural living, and the
nagging enervation will vanish!

Haphazard living is the true reason why you feel dragged-out,
weak, worn, prematurely old, and full of aches and pains ...
headed for the human scrap heap.

When you live as God and nature intended you to live,
you start to rejuvenate yourself.

Most people think they can attempt to break all nature's good and
just laws of Healthful Living. How very wrong they are ... you
cannot ever break a natural law. It will break you. You may
think you can break all of the natural laws — then run to a doctor
to circumvent these natural laws and have a miracle performed
on you.

THE MIRACLE IS IN YOU

The human being craves sudden miracles. Not satisfied with the
actual achievements of Natural Nutrition, Exercise, and Fasting,
which are in themselves miraculous, he searches in the realm of
the unknown for manifestations that he cannot understand.

21

Following nature's great laws is too simple a procedure to follow. People who are full of miseries and premature aging want a quick, easy way to find health and youthfulness. JUST REMEMBER, YOU MUST EARN YOUR HEALTH! You cannot buy it. No one can give it to you. I have boundless energy, great power, wonderful strength, and radiant, vibrant health ... because I have studied Nature's Laws and follow them. Natural nutritional laws, the laws of self-purification, which by fasting and keeping the circulation free-flowing and normal and the skin and muscle tone active by exercise, lead to agelessness.

HAVE YOU ANY HARMFUL HABITS YOU WISH TO OVERCOME?

Do you eat salt and salty foods? Do you drink coffee? Use tobacco? Alcohol? Use refined white sugar, or products with this devitalized material in it? What devitaminized and demineralized foods are dragging you down and enervating you? Is your will-power weak or strong? Who is the boss of your body? The bad habits? Or does your mind control your appetites. REMEMBER, FLESH IS DUMB! It cannot think for you. Only by positive thinking can you overcome the bad habits that dumb flesh craves. If you really crave Super Power, Glorious Health, Uncanny Strength, Tremendous Nerve Force, and a body you will be proud of, start working with Nature today and not against her!

Fasting is the key which unlocks Nature's storehouse of energy. It reaches every cell in the body, the inner organs, and generates the Life Forces. No one can do it for you ... it is a personal duty that only YOU can perform. No one can eat for you. And I believe that 99% of all human suffering is caused by wrong and unnatural eating. The efficiency of any machine depends upon the quality and amount of generating power it is given. And that goes for the human machine.

People blame everything on earth except food, as the cause of their physical miseries and premature aging. Whey they are suffering is a mystery to them. The average person does not know how horribly unclean the inside of the body is, caused by years and years of overeating, eating when not really hungry, and in many cases, wrong-eating of dead, devitalized foods. Which all helps in building up internal poisons and toxic wastes in their body.

Put the person who brags that he "Enjoys Perfect Health" on a complete, exclusive, distilled water-fast for 5 or 6 days. His breath will become putrid, his tongue will have a rancid, foul-smelling, white coating. His urine will be dark and evil-smelling This definitely proves that his whole body is filled up with decayed uneliminated materials brought in exclusively by eating.

The continual, accumulated, increasing, foul body-poison is his buried or latent, "unknown misery" and when Nature wants to get rid of it by any kind of an "explosion" commonly known as sickness ... man looks for anything fast and easy to get rid of his troubles, except to stop eating and fast.

FASTING — A NATURAL INSTINCT

Sickness is Nature's way of indicating that you are filled with toxic wastes and internal poison. Dead people do not have miseries. It is only when you are alive and have "Vital Power" that you have physical problems. In fasting, you are working with Nature to help expel the wastes and poisons you have accumulated in your body. Every animal in the wilderness knows this. Fasting is the only method an animal has to help overcome any physical trouble that befalls him. This is pure animal instinct. We humans have lived so long in this soft civilization that we have lost the instinct to fast when troubles occur in our bodies.

You may have experienced in your life a time when you were suffering physically and felt no desire for food. Food even repulsed you ... kind but ignorant relatives or friends told you, you must "eat to keep up your strength". The very last thing you needed was food, because your subconscious mind was signaling you to stop eating. Nature wanted you to fast, so she could use your "Vital Power" to cleanse your body-house. The soft voice of Mother Nature is hard to hear and understand. By fasting, your extrasensory instinct becomes very keen. The fast sharpens the mind ... tunes you in with the gentle voice of nature. Fasting has made my inner mind alert. I know positively that my mind works sharper and better after each fast I take.

THE GREAT MASTERS FASTED

In the great city of Alexandria, Egypt, in times when it was the educational center of the world ... people had to fast for 40 days before they could enter and study with the master of that time. Jesus fasted for forty days, and Buddha, took long fasts, so did Ghandi! All the great spiritual leaders since history began have had great confidence in the power of fasting ... not only to improve the physical body ... but to have a keener understanding of the power higher than ourselves ... to create a greater mental power! Prove it to yourself. See how much sharper and more alert your mind becomes after a fast ... notice how quickly you acquire facts. Notice how much more your mind absorbs while reading.

★ ★ ★ ★ ★

He that never eats too much will never be lazy.

★

The doors of wisdom are never shut.
— Ben Franklin

Take time
for **12** things

1 ***Take time to Work—***
    it is the price of success.

2 ***Take time to Think—***
    it is the source of power.

3 ***Take time to Play—***
    it is the secret of youth.

4 ***Take time to Read—***
    it is the foundation of knowledge.

5 ***Take time to Worship—***
    *it is the highway of reverance and washes the
    dust of earth from our eyes.*

6 ***Take time to Help and Enjoy Friends—***
    it is the source of happiness.

7 ***Take time to Love—***
    it is the one sacrament of life.

8 ***Take time to Dream—***
    it hitches the soul to the stars.

9 ***Take time to Laugh—***
    it is the singing that helps with life's loads.

10 ***Take time for Beauty—***
    it is everywhere in nature.

11 ***Take time for Health—***
    it is the true wealth and treasure of life.

12 ***Take time to Plan—***
    *it is the secret of being able to have time to
    take time for the first eleven things.*

---

*Every man is the builder of a temple called his body . . . We are all sculptors and
painters, and our material is our own flesh and blood and bones. Any nobleness
begins at once to refine a man's features, any meanness or sensuality to imbrute
them.*

— **Henry David Thoreau**

THE ENEMY WITHIN OUR BODIES

3

Victor Hugo poetically called the poison in our body "the serpent which is in man".

While this remark is poetic, it contains even more truth than poetry. I have come to regard autointoxication as my worst, grimmest foe in the fight for Agelessness and Longevity. It is even more devastating morally than physically. It is mind-poisoning as well as body-poisoning, and even after the energy of the body is regained, one has a lingering sense of the futility of all energy. One is inclined to say: "The best of life is behind me. What lies before is brief and burdensome. So many of my friends and relations have gone. Others say, my turn's coming. I've got a date with the undertaker, and maybe it's not so far off, either." These thoughts generate sad, depressing moods and are most unfriendly to Agelessness and Longevity.

But autointoxication itself is the greatest enemy of long living because it is so common and yet so little recognized. Those morbid moods, the worry, tensions, stresses, frustrations, nervousness, needless anxiety are foreign to a healthy state of the blood. You should always be optimistic, gay, happy, care-free, self-confident, and serene. Why is it that sometimes when fortune smiles her brightest, you are unhappy, mirthless, depressed, and ungrateful? Then again when things look their blackest, you are amazed at your buoyancy. The purity or impurity of your blood stream might explain that!

I want to live 120 years and more in prime physical condition - I love life! Each day of my life is a miracle - I hold life in the palm of my hand - I want to keep it - value it - treasure it and enjoy it every waking hour!

A DARK CLOUD OVER THE MIND

The worst of autointoxication is that it has been coming on for a matter of years. It takes water-fasting, good natural eating, and clean living habits to defeat it.

When these poisons are surging through your body, you are unreasonably pessimistic and unable to throw off your feeling of depression. The mockery of life comes home to you. Is it all worth while? ... Then one morning you awake your cheery self again. Though a bit battered, you have beaten off the foe. Newspapers, T.V., and radio all sell products that make promises to relieve you of that "half-alive" feeling. Which one do you take? Remember, there are no "short-cuts" to feeling your best, physically and mentally.

> You are punished by your bad habits of living! You are greatly rewarded by your good habits of living!

Old Mother Nature will not let you get away with abusing your body. You must pay a big price every time you insult your body with dead and devitalized foods. Of course, you could take some kind of "dope" to deaden your body, but you are living in a fool's paradise if you think you can eat any old thing and then swallow some kind of "dope" and get away with it. You pay a dear price every time you make a garbage can of your stomach! Your heart has suffered. Your arteries have suffered. Your little spell of autointoxication has done something towards shortening your life. Every attack leaves its mark, and, for this reason, it is something to be dreaded. Never let your blood stream become poisoned. Learn to defend yourself against autointoxication.

First, make it a habit to take a complete water-fast once a week of from 24 to 36 hours. And on the days you eat ... eat natural, unpoisoned foods. Let your mind rule your body. Flesh is dumb. You can feed your stomach anything. But now you are going to use commonsense, eat with intelligence. Always eat foods as close to nature as possible!

WHY KILL YOURSELF SO SOON?

Keep this firmly in mind. Autointoxication is our greatest enemy It is the root cause of all our major physical troubles, because they have their beginning in a poisoned blood stream. It is at the bottom of most of the troubles which affect the heart, liver, kidneys, joints, and arteries. The poisoned life stream has more to do with premature old age than all other causes put together. To keep your blood pure is half the battle; yet you deliberately poison it. You often overcharge your stomach, giving it a new job before it has finished digesting the old.

You have been taught that you should eat at regular times ... whether you are hungry or not ... it is mealtime, so you stuff yourself ... this is a terrible way to live ... it is wrong ... out-of-date scientifically with all the new discoveries of natural nutrition.

I recently took a voyage for a number of days ... they fed passengers an early morning breakfast in their staterooms ... then an hour or so later they filled them with a tremendous breakfast of bacon, ham and eggs, hot rolls, toast, jam, jelly, fried potatoes, and gallons of coffee, then a snack on deck at 11 A.M. A big lunch was served at 1 P.M., afternoon tea with gooey pastries at 4 P.M., a whopper of a big dinner at 7 P.M., and at 11 P.M. a big buffet dinner. Believe it or not, we buried 9 people at sea in a few weeks. All died by self-poison ... Autointoxication! When you overeat, you encourage fermentation and putrefaction, create discord of harmony, thus inviting millions of microbes to breed in your intestines.

LIFE IS SLOW SUICIDE

From the cradle you start to do yourself in, and while you are lightheartedly lopping off the years at the beginning of existence, you are cheerfully chopping them off in chunks at the end. Blissfully unconscious, you burn your candle at both ends. Sometimes you even try to burn it in the middle. We are dying before our time because we lack a sense of the sanity of living.

There is little doubt that any person born with a sound constitution according to the science of health, should without difficulty reach the 120 year mark!

Why not? There are no such things as old age diseases. There is only one thing that can kill you and that is some fatal disease. Now, reason with me ... if you live from childhood, eating scientifically ... fasting one day a week, and several times a year for periods of from 7 to 10 days ... how is it possible to get a fatal disease?

Children of our present age are being fed all wrong. First, most mothers cannot nurse their young babies. They lack the internal vitality to produce the greatest food in the world for their young ... Mothers' Milk. Their babies are bottle-fed ... and are given baby food out of bottles and cans, loaded with refined white flours, refined white sugar, and generously full of deadly salt.

The abuse of the physical machine of the modern child is started at birth. And premature breakdown is inevitable.

★ ★ ★ ★ ★

Nine men in ten are suicides.   — Ben Franklin

Look about you if you want enlightenment on the subject of health. Every day there are 25 million Americans critically ill in thousands of hospitals spread across our country from coast to coast. 300,000 doctors are kept frantically busy trying to patch the desperately sick people in our country! 80,000 dentists cannot do one-tenth of all the dental work that is required in the mouths of the average American!

I find most children's mouths are filled with decay and cavities before they are seventeen ... many children are forced to have dentures before they are twenty. We are a hopelessly sick, sick nation. We are brainwashed to believe we are a healthy and vital U.S.A. But the facts and figures do not lie. And even if you don't overeat, the food you eat is of the wrong kind. It is acid in reaction, instead of alkaline. Yet a little knowledge of physiology, diet, and fasting could save you. Ignorance is a worse enemy than indulgence. You can't be a walking germ-factory and expect to live the good life.

OUT OF THE GREASY FRYING PAN

I was reared in the South, in Virginia. My diet was terrible. Ninety percent of my food was prepared in the frying pan: fried chicken, fried ham, bacon, potatoes, pork chops, and fried meats of all kinds. I ate heavy cream and flour gravies, hot biscuits and plenty of pies, cakes, and jellies. When I look back, I see I suffered for years from autointoxication and didn't know it. Despite a horror of drugs, I let myself be doped by the poisons within me. Rarely was I entirely free of them, and the average health I enjoyed was far from the radiant health that was my heritage.

I usually slept ten hours a night instead of eight, and the excess was largely the deep stupor of autointoxication. Even after a long night of sleep, I seldom woke up to begin the day refreshed and eager. Usually I'd be dull and peevish. I had a bitter taste in my mouth. Often I arose reluctantly, feeling existence a bore, rather than a boon.

Most people are not really living ... they are existing. They are so full of toxic poisons that life is an effort. Few people rise eagerly, impatient to resume the adventure of living.

Let us look on our bedrooms as recharge areas where we are required to spend a certain length of time in sleep to recharge our life batteries. Let us make our bedrooms charming and restful — but do not let their brightness blind us to the beauty of the dawn. Let us get golden inspiration by seeing the sun start on its daily round, as it rises out of the eastern sky. During the early morning hours you always seem to get more accomplished — so try and cultivate early morning rising — you can if you put your mind to it --- then in the afternoon — you will have some time for a little "cat-nap" — seeing you got an early start on the day with early rising.

I can plainly see why so many people use stimulants such as tobacco, alcohol, coffee, tea, cola drinks and "pep pills" to try and fight the desperate moods of melancholy and frustration caused by autointoxication.

I could go on for pages depicting the woes of toxic infection. My blood was poisoned, my life stream plugged at its source. No-. one would deliberately foul a pure stream, yet, consistently, I polluted the most precious part of my life — my blood stream.

OUTWITTING ACIDOSIS

Yes, it has taken me all these years of research and study to discover the great fact ... that the blood stream should be alkaline. Yet, with most of us, it is an acid reaction. From headache and indigestion, to pimples and common cold, most of our miseries arise from acidosis — and it is because of autointoxication. When the life stream is so polluted, how can we defend ourselves against the germs of maladies that only await a chance to gain a footing? We carefully prepare the ground for the microbe, invite it to make itself at home, and let it have the jolliest of good times at our imbecile expense.

Now if you are as ignorant as I was, you will ask: "What can I do to counteract this supposed acidity? How can I cleanse my blood?" The answer is: "By supplying it with alkaline — forming constituents." On the first sign of autointoxication you should go on a three- to four-day water-fast and, after the fast, switch to an alkaline-forming diet, and at all times you should avoid acid-forming foods. "But what are alkaline-forming foods?" you ask. Generally speaking; Raw fruits and vegetables ... made into salads ... along with leafy, green, cooked vegetables. Three-fifths of your diet should be composed of fruits and vegetables. ... both raw and cooked. Always eat a raw vegetable salad or fresh fruit before you eat any meal. The alkaline-forming foods are the most important to your body. Some of you will say "raw fruits and vegetables do not agree with me". That is because you are on the acid side ... and when you eat the alkaline foods, they start to clean-up the toxic dirt that is in your blood stream. So, you brush off the whole subject, and use the weak excuse that certain fruits and vegetables do not agree with you ... they agree with you, but your toxic body does not agree with them.

★ ★ ★ ★ ★

Don't injure your system by over-feeding it.
Over-eating will kill you long before your time.

RAW FRUITS AND VEGETABLES — NATURE'S CLEANSERS

When you get a reaction from certain raw fruits and vegetables ... remember these are cleansing and purifying foods. Use a small amount until you can reduce the toxic poison ... your weekly 24-hour fast is going to get rid of a lot of your body wastes. And, if you have the intestinal strength to fast for 3 to 7 days, most of your troubles of food disagreeing with you will be over. What are the acid-forming foods? Chiefly sugar, sugar products, coffee, tea, alcohol, grains, meats, and fish.

No doubt the idea of tabooing even a portion of the latter will dismay you, but if you want to live agelessly you must do many things that dismay you at first. Eventually you will be dismayed at your dismay. Often a new task is difficult because you think it is. Tackle it with the idea that it is easy and it becomes easy. Living on a diet composed mainly of fruit, vegetables, salads, nuts, and seeds is not difficult. No one will deny that fruits are luscious. Salads may be had in great variety. The list of vegetables is long and diversified. All the nuts and seeds are nourishing and tasty ... Raw peanuts (lightly roasted) pecans, almonds, walnuts, sunflower seeds, sesame seeds, etc. are delicious and nutritious. You need not confine yourself to these particular foods but, if you have a tendency to acidosis, you should see that, together with fasting, they predominate in your diet.

If you eat meat, it should be only two or three times weekly. And on the least symptom of feeling bad, you should get back to the alkaline diet quickly. The signs are many — slight headaches, dizziness, specks in the vision, bitterness in the mouth, physical slackness, and mental blockage. Of course, these merely denote a bilious attack, but again the disorder may be more deep-seated. If you think it is only your liver, you may merely cut out the fats and flesh foods, but that is not enough. You should cut out the sugars and starches, too. That is to say, you should take them in their natural form of fruit and vegetables. The little protein you need, you can get from nuts and seeds.

Prudently assume, then, that your condition is one of incipient autointoxication, for it is rarely absent in some slight form. If you feel your energy at a low ebb, and you are not up to par, go on a short fast for from 36 hours to three or four days. Drink nothing but clear, fresh water ... I prefer distilled water (will tell you more about that later).

You will experience a craving for food. But it is not an actual hunger ... it is the reflexes of the body that are accustomed to being fed at certain intervals. Again let me state ... FLESH IS DUMB ... it has all kinds of cravings ... but you must be the master — you must control the entire body with the mind. I can readily admit that fasting takes immense determination and will power ... it is a battle of mind over matter.

I remember very well my first four-day fast. It was while I was under the guidance of the famous Dr. A. Rollier of Leysin, Switzerland. I was battling for my life with tuberculosis, and I had been at the sanitarium for over a year. Dr. Rollier told me it was going to be a great experience for me — and it surely was. The good doctor told me to study my urine each day. So, each day I took a specimen of my urine and kept it in a bottle. I carefully put it on a shelf in my bedroom and I would look at the specimens each day. As the urine would cool and settle I could see the great amount of foreign matter that was leaving my body.

NOTE: NO ONE SHOULD FAST WHO HAS A DISEASE UNLESS UNDER THE STRICT SUPERVISION OF A DOCTOR or someone who has had long experience in the science of fasting. As soon as I finished the fast, I was placed on a highly alkaline diet with an abundance of fresh fruits, raw vegetables, and cooked vegetables. In about two weeks after the fast, I experienced a sense of exhilaration and well-being that I had never known before in my entire life.

From that time on my health and vitality grew in leaps and bounds. That was not my only fast under Dr. Rollier's supervision ... he started me then on the 24-hour fast weekly, and, in the next nine months, put me on a 7-day, 14- and 21-day fast. Between fasts I was fed on an alkaline diet.

KEEP YOUR STOMACH ALKALINE

Because acidosis is more of a negative than a positive ill, you should beware of it. Have you never said: "Oh, I'm a little off-color; loss of pep; a bit blue for no real reason. Everyone has his off-days. It seems to be a part of life". Nothing of the kind. You can maintain yourself in a state of consistent good health, not spasmodic good health. You can come to consider your body, a fine machine, that with proper care will never go wrong.

Check acidosis, then, at its first suspicion of a sign. A grayish tongue, a snappish temper, a flushing of the face ... do not look on these as too trivial to heed. They are signs of danger. Perhaps today they may not amount to much, but tomorrow they will be more insistent. Acidosis is insidious and accumulative in its action, and it is today, not tomorrow, that you should begin to defend yourself. For life is self-defense. Your adversary has you at a disadvantage, and what you lack in stamina you must make up for in strategy. You are fighting a losing fight. You will be knocked out in the end, but whether the match lasts ten rounds or twenty entirely depends on you.

Beware then of acidosis and all of the evils it invites. Apart from asking for trouble from invading germs, it will, if chronic, lead to a permanently high blood pressure and its consequent doom of arteriosclerosis (hardening of the arteries). Thus, the chain is complete: overacid dietary — autointoxication — high blood pressure — stiff arteries — premature death. So, even if they call you a food crank, don't be too sensitive. Remember, it's your funeral. Let the so-called 100% normal people sneer. Perhaps the last laugh will be yours. At the first danger signs, switch from the potato to the tomato, from cheese to fruit. If you cannot keep your blood neutral, keep it alkaline. But on no account let it get acid. The danger is greater because it is not obvious. Few realize that they suffer from mild, yet chronic, acidosis, and that sooner or later it will mean discomfort, disease, and untimely death.

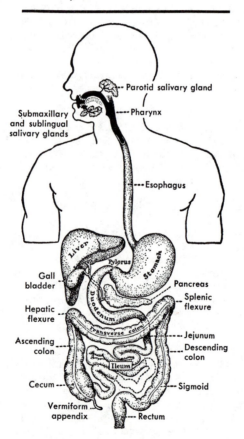

The relationships of the different parts of the digestive system. Only a small part of the small intestine shown.

4

TOXIC ACID
CRYSTALS
CAN CEMENT YOUR MOVABLE JOINTS. MAKE YOU STIFF, AND FILL YOU FULL OF MISERY. FIGHT DEADLY ACID CRYSTALS BY
FASTING

Stand on any street corner and watch the average person hobble along. The feet, knees, hips, spine, and head seem to be cemented...there is no free-swinging movement in their loco-motion. Let's look at their feet. They seem to pick up their feet heavily and lay them down flatly...their knees seem to be completely cemented and stiff...there is little movement in the swinging motion in the hips, their spines are rigid and so are their heads. All of the elasticity and resiliency in the body seems to have gone out of what should be a free-swinging body.

CEMENT INSTEAD OF LUBRICATION
FOR MOVABLE JOINTS

Between the movable joints of every bone in the human body, nature at one time placed an abundant supply of a lubrication known as synovial fluid. Take a look at a youngster who is, say 10 years of age, and see the easy movement of every mov-able joint in the body.

W H Y ?

I know what your answer would be... "This child is only 10 years of age...I am 66. I can't have the freedom of motion of my joints as child of 10 does." My answer to you is... "WHY CAN'T YOU? Years have nothing to do with the amount

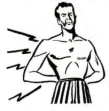

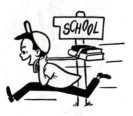

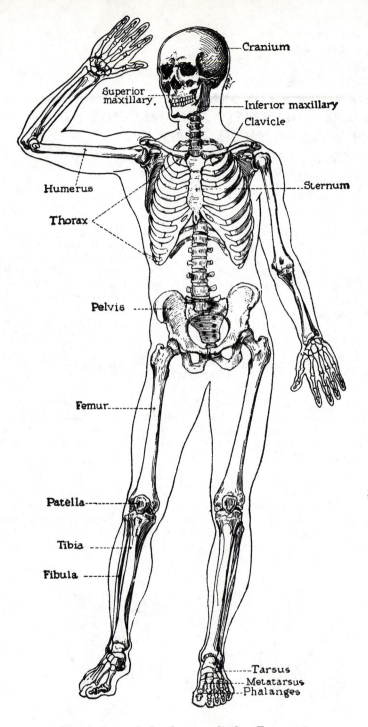

Cranium

Superior maxillary.

Inferior maxillary

Clavicle

Sternum

Humerus

Thorax

Pelvis

Femur

Patella

Tibia

Fibula

Tarsus

Metatarsus

Phalanges

The bones of the human body. Front view.

of synovial fluid that makes the joints move freely and easily. There is just one thing that cements your movable joints and that is TOXIC ACID CRYSTALS. "

Age is not toxic, because you live 40 - 50 - 60 or 70 years, there should be no diminishing of the supply of synovial fluid due to your calendar years.

TOXIC ACID CRYSTALS CAN CEMENT YOUR MOVABLE JOINTS

I am a man of 85 at the time of writing this book, and I pride myself on having the most flexible joints of any man, regardless of age. I perform difficult yoga postures with ease while standing on my head. Few people in the world can do this regardless of age. Now, Nature does not stiffen and cement one person's joints and yet allow me to have the flexibility of a boy of 10.

HOW YOU BUILD THE TOXIC ACID CRYSTALS IN YOUR BODY

There are four great eliminative systems in our body that get rid of the poisons created in our daily living. By Nature, we eat food, we drink liquids, and we breathe air. Most humans eat too much food, eating by habit rather than by hunger...they have been brainwashed to believe that they must have meals by the clock. I know from long experience as a Physical Therapist, that people with these grotesque shapes, have not been able to burn up these so-called regular meals. They have been conditioned to eat breakfast whether they have a real hunger or not, so they load in ham, bacon, eggs, hot cakes, doughnuts, toast, jelly, marmalade, sweet rolls, fried potatoes, waffles, pork sausage, coffee, tea, chocolate, and dry and cooked cereals.

The body does not have enough "Vital Force" to masticate, digest, assimilate and eliminate these heavy breakfasts. There is always a toxic residue left, and where does this toxic residue go? It is concentrated and crystalized and finds its way into the movable joints in the body. It's a slow process that few sense until the joints start to give trouble. It takes years and years of wrong eating to bring about the heavy concentration of acid crystals in the movable joints...but when these calcium-like spurs attach themselves on the joints and calcified substances replace the synovial fluid, then pains and aches are felt in the movable joints of the body.

The first place they attack is the feet. The foot has more movable bones than any other part of the body. There are 26 movable bones in each foot. The force of gravity sends the toxic crystals down into the feet. Gradually the feet and the ankles start to

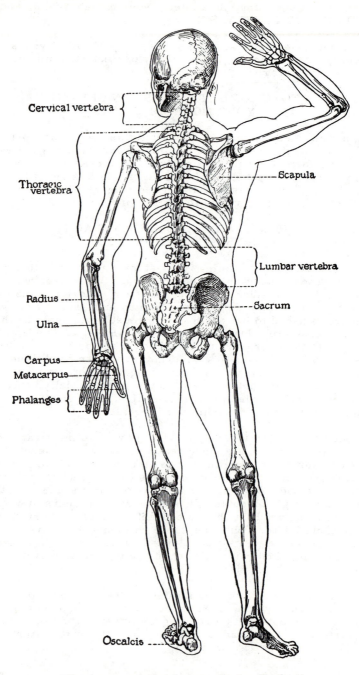

Cervical vertebra

Thoracic
vertebra

Scapula

Lumbar vertebra

Radius

Sacrum

Ulna

Carpus

Metacarpus

Phalanges

Oscalcis

The bones of the human body. Back view.

stiffen, because the toxic acid crystals are taking over and re-
placing the lubrication in the joints of the feet. So instead of the
feet being flexible, they harden and cement. They tire easily...
they ache, burn, and give a tremendous amount of physical
misery.

From the feet and ankles, the toxic acid crystals move up causing
many people to suffer with pains in the knees. Time marches on,
and so does the deterioration of the joints. Now the toxic crystals
have moved into the great movable joints of the hips and you notice by the way people move their hips that they are stiff and feeling pain.

LOWER BACK PAINS - THE CURSE OF MANKIND

Few people escape an aching or stiff back. Watch middle-aged
people bend over, see the agony on their faces when they straight-
en up. Day after day they cry out in anguish, "Oh, My Aching
Back"...but the toxic acid crystals don't stop in the lower back,
they go up into the spine, in the shoulder blades, in the shoulder
joints, in the neck, elbow joints, and even creeping into the wrists
and fingers. Some people are so full of toxic acid crystals that
they cannot close their fists. They all seem to blame one thing...
"All my aches and pains are due to the fact that I am getting old".

DON'T YOU BELIEVE IT. These acid crystals are poisons that
stayed in your body and cemented themselves in the movable
joints of the body. Billions of pain-killer pills are used by the
American public to get relief from aching joints. Thousands of
people seek hot mineral baths to get relief. Many, many treatments are used for the relief of their miseries. I have no cure
for stiffened joints. I want it definitely understood that I am not
prescribing for aching and stiff joints. But I maintain that there
are roads to relief.

FASTING FOR PURIFICATION

When you fast for 24-hours or 36-hours or from 3- to 10-days,
the healing power starts to work in your body. I have told you,
over and over, that the power to cleanse, purify, and renovate is
within your body. This power has always been in your body. When
you go on a complete distilled water-fast, the "Vital Power" in
your body that would ordinarily be used to masticate, digest,
assimilate, and eliminate food is used to purify your body. That
is what fasting is...deep internal cleansing - a physiological
rest to build "Vital Power".

Now, say you are a person of 60, and you have been eating 3
meals daily, whether you were hungry or not, and you have
allowed toxic acid crystals to get into the movable joints of the

body...it is going to take time for Nature and the power within your body to break down the toxic crystals that you have accumulated over the years.

THE CRIPPLE WHO REBUILT HIMSELF

I remember a Mr. Evans who came to me about 10 years ago. He hobbled painfully into my office. A well-known doctor in California had given him a prescription which read "Physical Therapy as prescribed".

I am a licensed Physical Therapist - licensed by the State Board of Medical Examiners of the State of California.

This man's story is one of millions of humans in our country. He had never been educated to know how to care for his wonderful body, but had been conditioned to eat 3 meals per day and eat anything that agreed with him. Now, I have told you several times in this manuscript that "Human Flesh is Dumb". You can put anything in your stomach at any hour that you are awake. You can get up in the morning and fill up on cereal, ham and eggs, fried potatoes, and toast, and wash it down with 5 cups of coffee, but you must take the consequences of eating habits like this. First, your body has to earn its food by the sweat of your brow, and that means you only eat food according to your physical activity, but here was a man who was eating as he did when he was a young active boy on the farm, and slowly his joints were loaded with toxic crystals that were now pressing on nerves causing him agonizing pain.

He wanted an easy way out of his misery, but I told him very truthfully that it had taken him a long time of wrong eating and bad habits of living to get in this wretched condition, and that it would take fasting and a good diet with plenty of alkaline foods to relieve these pains. He was an intelligent man and saw the truth of my philosophy. I started him on a 3-day distilled water fast and following the fast I had him eat only fresh fruit for breakfast...a raw vegetable combination salad for lunch, with 2 cooked vegetables. In the evening, I had him eat grated carrots, grated cabbage, and one cooked vegetable. I took him off all animal products, meat, fish, eggs, and dairy products. I eliminated salt, all grains, all legumes, such as beans, peas, rice, and lentils. Every day I had him take a 10-minute hot bath, bringing the water up to 104 degrees, using a bath thermometer, I gave him a walking schedule starting with 3 blocks the first day, and every third day I would add another block to his walking schedule until I had him walking 5 miles a day.

It is well these days to be health-minded. Health is real and earnest, for it is actually life in duration and abundance. It is the opposite of the stiff, hobbling, sick-bed and the wheel chair.

VICTORY WON BY FASTING, DIET AND EXERCISE

Every week he had a 36-hour water fast, and as the days and weeks rolled on, I gave him one 7-day fast and one 10-day fast. In one year you would hardly recognize this man, his family, his friends were amazed at his transformation. His joints became flexible, and although he hadn't swum for years, he joined the Y.M.C.A. and swam two or three days a week. He hadn't ridden a bicycle for years, yet now he purchased one and rode miles and miles at a time. He and his wife took up dancing, and in a year he was winning dancing contests. The stiffness left him... he took up the piano and became a very good piano player. Mr. Evans is growing younger as he is growing older. Gone are his miseries. This was all accomplished by himself. I only helped him help himself. I never laid my hands on his body. As a Physical Therapist, I laid out his program of natural living. Today he fasts every week from 24 to 36 hours without fail. Four times a year, winter, spring, fall and summer he takes a 10 day complete fast. His lively steps are that of a man 20 years of age...his movements are quick and accurate. He didn't do all this in a day, in a week or a month. It took time for him to break the toxic acid crystals that were tormenting him.

What Mr. Evans did you can do! The body is self-repairing and self-healing, and self-maintaining. All you have to do is live by the laws of Nature, and Nature will reward you with the joy of living.

Fasting is an important part of a program for banishing toxic acid crystals from the movable joints of the body. You and only you know how free your joints are of this premature aging toxic material. Start today on your first 24-hour, distilled-water fasting - you be the judge what effects fasting will have on the many movable joints of your body. At this very second, roll your head round and round - do you hear the grating, grinding sound? The grinding sound you hear is the toxic acid crystals that have alkalified themselves on the first bone of your spine - the Atlas. Your 24-hour or your 7-day fast will not eliminate all the toxic acid crystals from your Atlas, but the work of body purification will be started. Fast one day a week - in one year you have fasted 52 days - in that time the "Vital Power" of your body has dissolved a large amount of acid crystals from your joints.

NATURE WORKS SLOWLY - BUT SURELY

Each time you fast you will notice more freedom in every movable joint in your body. The feeling of agelessness will replace that tight, stiff, aging feeling. Once again you will feel loose in every movable joint of the body. You will have fasting and eating natural food to thank for your "New Youthful Feeling".

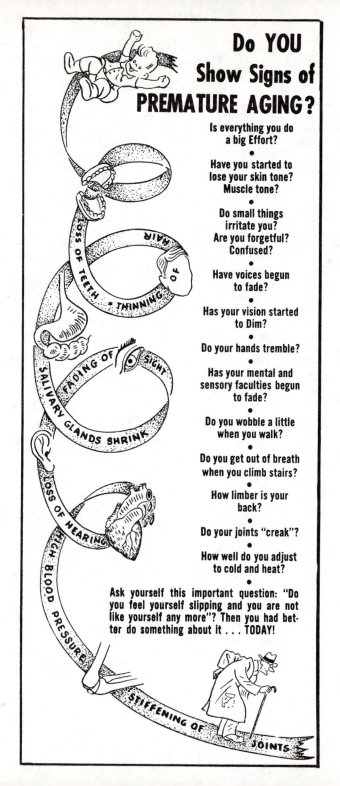

Do YOU Show Signs of PREMATURE AGING?

Is everything you do a big Effort?

•

Have you started to lose your skin tone? Muscle tone?

•

Do small things irritate you? Are you forgetful? Confused?

•

Have voices begun to fade?

•

Has your vision started to Dim?

•

Do your hands tremble?

•

Has your mental and sensory faculties begun to fade?

•

Do you wobble a little when you walk?

•

Do you get out of breath when you climb stairs?

•

How limber is your back?

•

Do your joints "creak"?

•

How well do you adjust to cold and heat?

•

Ask yourself this important question: "Do you feel yourself slipping and you are not like yourself any more"? Then you had better do something about it . . . TODAY!

SCIENTIFIC FASTING

5

EXPLAINED WITH FULL DIRECTIONS

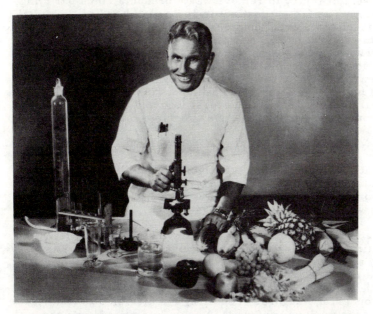

Bragg - Specialist In Nutrition And Life Extension

Fasting has been practiced by man and animal since the beginning of time. Primitive man had no other method of healing except fasting. Ages ago, man would fast when he got hurt or when he was ill, because fasting was part of his instinct for self-preservation. Along with fasting, he used herbs from the field and forest as a tonic and an antiseptic.

I believe that fasting is Mother Nature's greatest remedy! For as we will see, properly-conducted fasts purify the body, restoring it to health after everything else has failed.

In over 70 years of supervising fasts, I have seen things happen to people who were ready for the human scrapheap that could be called "miraculous". Fasting is not only the oldest method of fighting physical problems, but the best of all remedies as well, because it has no side-effects. It is the most natural, original process of purifying the body.

The instinct that leads us to fast when the body is sick or wounded resides in the cells of every living being. The reason why sick or wounded animals refuse to eat is because the instinct of self-preservation takes away their hunger so they will not eat. In this way the vital energy (which would otherwise have to be used in the digestion of food) is concentrated at the seat of injury to remove waste products, thus purifying the body. The fasting instinct is so powerful and of such vital importance that, even though semi-civilized man has strayed from the natural path, he is still greatly influenced by this wonderful saving scheme of nature! And if he would obey the silent voice of this infallible, natural instinct, and stop eating when natural hunger has been withdrawn, he would soon get well if he is sick, and would never get sick once he recovered his health, provided he ate natural food and lived in a natural environment...And lived a sane, sensible, natural life.

FASTING IS AS OLD AS MAN

Inasmuch as the infallible intelligence of the living organism with-draws the sensation of hunger when there is an excess of food, or when the body has been wounded, the desire to fast begins when either of these things happen.

We read in ancient history that fasting has been practiced since time immemorial by the religious people of the East, and by ancient civilizations. They practiced fasting not only for the recovery of health and preservation of youth, but for spiritual illumination as well. Accordingly, we see the great philosopher, Pythagoras, requiring his disciples to undertake a fast of forty days, before they could be initiated into the mysteries of his occult philosophical teachings. He claimed that only through a forty-day fast could the minds of his disciples be sufficiently purified and clarified to understand the profound teachings of the mysteries of life.

As it was in the old days, fasting will not only purify the body and help restore it to well-being, but could have a great effect on the mental and spiritual part of man.

FASTING AWAKENS THE MIND

In my own personal life, as well as in the lives of many of my students who have been conscientious and persistent in their fasting program, great mental and spiritual doors have been opened! If I read a book today, my mind retains what I read as clearly as if the book were in front of me, that it, I have a photographic mind. Hundreds of my students write that they too, have developed a keen photographic mind. After a fast of from one to three days, you will notice that a dark cloud has been lifted out of your mind. You can think more logically, and you can come to decisions quickly. What was once a great problem becomes trivial. After a fast, you seem to fear nothing any more, and things you worried about are solved easily by your purified mind.

In my personal life, I have developed a keen extrasensory perception. I can find solutions for many problems that once caused me many hours of anxiety and nerve-exhausting worrying.

My fasting program has developed an inner peaceful tranquillity of mind, and I feel more serene and at peace with myself and the world with my continued fasting program. As you purify your body and mind, you seem to come closer to a POWER HIGHER THAN YOURSELF! This inner-strength, this inner-power, makes you a positive-thinking person.

The memory becomes sharp as a razor's edge. You can remember names, places, and instances that go back many years. You have a better capacity for self-education. Education is not a preparation for life, but education is life itself! To grow mentally and spiritually is the greatest goal we humans can have on this earth. So fasting works three ways... you purify your body physically, mentally and spiritually and therefore enjoy super-vitality and super-health! Your mind becomes like a sponge which can absorb new facts and knowledge! Greatest of all is the inner peacefulness and spiritual tranquillity that make life worth living. Through fasting you find "Peace of Mind", the greatest and rarest boon of modern life.

BIBLICAL PATRIARCHS FASTED

We know that in ancient times the patriarchs of the Bible fasted frequently. Moses, Elijah, David, and others fasted for as long as forty days. We know that Christ fasted forty days before he began to teach the great truths of Life. We read in the Bible that Christ sent forth his disciples, saying to them: "Heal the sick, cleanse the leper, raise the dead, cast out devils, freely ye have received, freely give." At the same time, Christ knew that there were dangers awaiting those who dared to bring truth to the people. Therefore, Christ warned his disciples in these words: "Behold! I send you forth as sheep in the midst of wolves: be ye therefore wise as serpents and harmless as doves." (Matthew, Chapter 10:8, 16.)

As in the olden days, there are dispensers of gloom, fear, and destruction when the subject of fasting is brought up today. I have heard people discuss how unscientific fasting is and when I asked them if they had ever fasted, they gave me a definite answer "NEVER".

These dispensers of gloom still cling to the old idea that you must eat to keep up your strength, and that when you stop eating, you collapse. This is far from the truth! A few days of discomfort may occur during fasting which only happen because we are creatures of habit. If we are able to surmount the first 3 days of fasting, then it becomes a pleasure. You lose your appetite, you have no craving for food, therefore you have a tremendous amount of energy. Of course, if you are loaded with toxic poisons, fasting will flush these toxic poisons out of the body, and you will feel a little uncomfortable, but these are momentary experiences and should cause no concern. This means only that fasting is working for you. You know you are fasting to purify the body of the morbid toxic poisons and waste that you have accumulated. When you feel a little uncomfortable, you can say to yourself, "This is only temporary. This will pass as soon as these old toxins are flushed out of my body". And what a wonderful reward for the small amount of discomfort you may have had by fasting.

Your eyes become brighter, all the natural senses of the body seem to be sharper! After a fast your food tastes better and the fruits and the vegetables taste so marvelous, because of this new re-vitilized taste sense! Your body seems to be tireless, and you will sleep like a baby after a fast. There are so many rewards from a fast that only a person who has actually fasted can truly realize the great benefits that are achieved.

DON'T BE A SLAVE TO FOOD

Most humans are slaves to food; they must have breakfast, lunch and dinner at regular meal-hours every day, year-in and year-out. They eat whether they are hungry or not, and the poor body is burdened with over-nutrition and usually poor nutrition at that! No wonder we have so many physical wrecks! One of the greatest nutritional teachers in the world, Professor Arnold Ehret, said, "Life is a tragedy of nutrition". How true is the old trite saying, "Man digs his grave with his knife and fork". Many people never give their stomachs a rest ... they continually give the digestive and eliminating function an over-burden of food and this overburden means that the functions of digestion and elimination become so overworked and so exhausted that they simply collapse. The entire body becomes enervated.

After a fast, you will find you will not need nearly as much food as you have been accustomed to eating! The fast will shrink your stomach and you will feel better, look better, and have more vitality on one-half the food intake you were accustomed to in the past.

I am an active man physically. I put great physical demands on my body, and yet I eat only two light meals daily. I never snack between meals. Nibbling and compulsory eating has been eliminated from my life by my long years of the 24-hour weekly fast, and my fast of from 7 to 10 days, 3 or 4 times a year. After the fast, see how your eyes sparkle, and see the wonderful improvement in your skin-tone through fasting. Notice how much more energy and vitality you have, and, above all, notice the light-hearted song your heart sings, because your body is clean again ... it is not burdened with fighting toxic poisons. You have lifted a heavy burden from your blood-stream and the vital organs.

PLAN YOUR FASTING PROGRAM TODAY

So, if you want all these great benefits, be a strong positive person, plan a fasting program for yourself, and live strictly by it. Don't tell anyone you are going to fast, because the average person is ignorant of the facts on fasting and they are not qualified to criticize your fasting program. I never discuss my fasting program with people who have no knowledge of the wonders and miracles of fasting. Why should I discuss it with them? They are still full of the same old fears held by the average person; that if they miss a few meals, they will starve to death. So be intelligent enough not to tell your family what you are doing. You will simple get a lot of worthless advice. Many times while I am fasting for a week, I carry on my daily duties. I conduct large lecture campaigns and I reveal to no one that I am on a complete fast. Fasting is a very personal thing ... it is something that belongs to you, and not to your relatives and your friends! If you have faith in it, that is all that is necessary. You are putting faith in Nature's oldest and most respected way of purifying, renovating, and rejuvenating the body!

YOUR MIND MUST RULE YOUR BODY IF YOU ARE TO FAST SUCCESSFULLY

Remember what I have told you, "FLESH IS DUMB". It has no intelligence or reasoning power.

If, after reading this manuscript, you are convinced, without any reservations, that a fasting program is going to elevate you to greater heights of living, then your mind becomes the master of your flesh. Your mind must be stronger than the desires of your flesh, because your body has long been conditioned to have food put into it at various intervals of the day.

The average person gets up and eats breakfast whether he is hungry or not. The stomach does all the directing, the mind must tag along with the desires of the stomach ... so through reflex conditioning, the stomach expects food for breakfast. To me, breakfast is a worthless meal. The body has been at rest all night, it has not expended energy, so therefore, why should a person get up after the inactivity of sleep and put a big breakfast into the stomach. I have told you and I will reiterate for continuity of thought that, "YOU MUST EARN YOUR FOOD BY PHYSICAL ACTIVITY!"

Another reason why I am a believer and a follower of the non-breakfast plan, is because big breakfasts drain and exhaust most people of the energy that has been gathered by the night's sleep. In the morning, your energy ... physically, mentally, and spiritually ... should be the highest. With this new energy that the body has created, you can do great creative and physical work.

I have shown elementary school students, high school students, and college students that they can do their greatest studying early in the morning on an empty stomach. Most students eat an evening meal, which is their heaviest meal of the day, and then they try to study. What happens? It is a terrific effort to concentrate and study after eating a hugh dinner. It seems that the mind just will not work after a heavy meal, but give these same students a good night's rest, get them up early in the morning, and keep food out of them for 2 or 3 hours, and they will become geniuses. They will become brilliant. I have taught this to thousands of students all over the world. I have taught it to musicians, art students, sculpturers, and writers. This is the logical reason why I do not believe in a heavy breakfast. A heavy meal requires most of the total nerve energy of the body to handle the digestion, thus the mind becomes enervated, making people dull and sleepy ... meaning that the nerve energy is at its lowest ebb.

Let's look at it from another standpoint ... through long years of misinformation people have been told "breakfast is the most important meal of the day — it gives you the strength, the energy, and the vitality to do a hard morning's work, either physically or mentally". This is absolutely erroneous ... it is not a true scientific fact. When you eat a heavy breakfast, through reflex action you feel full and satisfied, but you do not gain strength. It takes hours for this food to be processed by the digestive system before you gain any energy or vitality from a big breakfast. Digestion is a most complicated process. Every item of food in the breakfast has to be broken down into fine chemical fragments, so that the cells of the body are fed.

★ ★ ★ ★ ★

Wisdom is the principal thing; therefore get wisdom: and with all thy getting get understanding. -- Proverbs 4:7

46

EARN YOUR FOOD BY EXERCISING

So you can plainly see that eating is a matter of conditioning and habit. I haven't eaten breakfast for over 50 years or more. I get up early in the morning, and if I am living at my Hollywood home, I get in my car and drive to our beautiful Griffith Park mountain trail, hike for several hours to the top of Mt. Hollywood and top it off by running down the mountain; or if I am at my beach home at Santa Monica, I take long hikes and runs on the beach. I am not only a summer bather, but I am a year-round ocean bather. At my desert home, I hike or ride my bicycle. After several hours of vigorous exercise, I return home and do my best creative work, planning my lectures, writing articles for health magazines, or writing books. Along towards 11 o'clock I have a piece of fruit, and about 12 o'clock I will eat my first meal of the day. I start with a large raw combination salad, the base of which is raw grated cabbage and carrots, then I will add other raw vegetables such as tomatoes, radishes, celery, beats, and top it off with half an avocado. I will eat one cooked yellow vegetable such as baked yam or carrots, one green vegetable, such as spinach, Swiss chard, kale, mustard greens, and some type of protein. I, of course, prefer nuts of all kinds, or seeds, such as sunflower seeds, pumpkin seeds or sesame seeds.

I have earned this meal by exercise and my body is now ready to send forth the digestive juices and the internal secretions to get all of the nourishment and energy out of this natural food. How wonderful this natural food tastes! The juices of the mouth and stomach are abundant, and elimination is absolutely perfect. In bowel elimination, outgo should equal intake.

This program of 12 meals a week, 2 meals per day, 6 days a week, (I fast one 24- or 36-hour period weekly) does not burden and exhaust the bowel eliminative powers of my body. On this program, I have educated my bowels to move immediately upon arising. I have a bowel evacuation within an hour after my lunch and within one hour after my evening meal.

The only exception I ever make eating between meals is to have some kind of luscious, juicy fruit. Sometimes, in midafternoon, I will have a firm juicy apple, or several slices of fresh pineapple. When melons are in season and the weather is warm, I find nothing more refreshing than a slice of melon, particularly red, ripe luscious watermelon.

Most people are sick or half-sick most of the time, and in my opinion I believe that they enervate themselves and exhaust themselves in trying to burn up all the extra food they consume.

EATING IS A SPORT IN AMERICA!

This is the reason why 65 to 70 percent of the people in this country are overweight. Eating has become a sport in America! People eat breakfast, eat at the coffee-break, eat at lunch, eat at their afternoon coffee-break. They eat a large dinner and, long before the big dinner is handled by the digestive apparatus, they are eating while watching T.V., and drinking alcohol, cola drinks, or coffee. No wonder they are constantly tired! It is because they enervate themselves by exhausting their vital power. Even the healthiest person only generates so much vital power every day and, if through eating habits or other bad habits, you exhaust the vital power, then there is not sufficient energy for the great work of mastication, digestion, metabolism, and elimination.

KEEP CLEAN INSIDE

What happens? There is not enough vital power to flush the waste out of the body so this waste piles and concentrates and that is how you build autointoxication. Your troubles and premature aging start right here!

Sickness and premature aging is no mystery. You are punished by your bad habits, not for them, but by them! If you keep stuffing food into your over-loaded digestive tract that cannot be handled, it only rots, putrifies, and poisons billions of your body cells. You are sick, weak, and prematurely old because you have not learned how to keep your body clean inside. The secret of health and long-life can be summed up in three words: "KEEP CLEAN INSIDE!" Sculpture these words of wisdom deep on the blackboard of your brain. Repeat them over and over again as an affirmation, "KEEP CLEAN INSIDE." FASTING is the one and only method of cleansing, purifying, and rejuvenating your body because it is Nature's Natural Method. Nobody can do it for you, it is a personal matter, it costs you nothing but a strong positive will-power! Remember Woe to the weak ... life is the survival of the fittest and fasting is a program of self-preservation.

ARE YOU READY TO FAST?

If you are convinced, without reservation, that fasting is going to be good for you, then you are ready. Remember, when you tell your conscious mind and your subconscious mind that you are going to fast for internal purity, you set things in motion for success. You have told every cell in your body that you believe that a fast is going to make you a better human. Every-one of your body cells are going to accept this command.

Start with a 24-hour distilled-water fast. Now during these 24-hours, you are going to put nothing into your stomach except distilled water. If you eat fruit with this, it is not a fast; it is a fruit diet. If you drink fruit or vegetable juices during this 24-hour period, it ceases to be a complete fast, but becomes either a vegetable or fruit diet. I want you to bear this in mind, a fast is nothing in the stomach except distilled water! Your first fast may be easy, or it may have some rough spots. You may fast from lunch to lunch, or dinner to dinner, as long as you abstain from food for 24 hours. If you are accustomed to coffee, tea, beer, or alcohol drinks, you might have reactions and one reaction generally appears in the form of a headache!

Why? Because the cells of your body have conditioned themselves to regular dosages of a stimulant. When you take the stimulant away from the nerves and the cells, there is bound to be a reaction, but remember this fast is going to help break that stimulant habit, because during the 24-hour, distilled-water fast, you are going to flush out of the body through the organs of elimination, many of the old buried residues of your pet poisons.

On a 24-hour fast, most people can carry on their regular duties, even though they may have a little discomfort, and there may be some turbulence in the stomach, but, all-in-all, it should go smoothly and successfully if you let your mind be the master of your flesh. You are giving the commands through the body from the higher brain cells. You are not going to be dragged down to the level of the lower cells of the stomach.

3 NEEDED HABITS

"There are three habits which with but one condition added, will give you every thing in the world worth having, and beyond which the imagination of man cannot conjure forth a single addition of improvement. These habits are:

   The Work Habit
   The Health Habit
   The Study Habit

If you are a man and have these habits, and also have the love of a woman who has these same habits, you are in paradise now and here, and so is she.

- Elbert Hubbard

Slow Me Down, Lord

Slow me down, Lord

Ease the pounding of my heart by the quieting of my mind.

Steady my hurried pace with a vision of the eternal reach of time.

Give me, amid the confusion of the day, the calmness of the everlasting hills.

Break the tensions of my nerves and muscles with the soothing music of the singing streams that live in my memory. Help me to know the magical, restoring power of sleep.

Teach me the art of taking minute vacations—of slowing down to look at a flower, to chat with a friend, to pat a dog, to read a few lines from a good book.

Slow me down, Lord, and inspire me to send my roots deep into the soil of life's enduring values that I may grow toward the stars of my greater destiny.

WHY I DRINK DISTILLED WATER EXCLUSIVELY

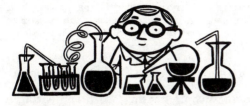

6

In this manuscript, when I refer to fasting, I constantly make the statement "Eat absolutely no food, no fruit or vegetable juices, and drink distilled water exclusively."

Distilled water is pure water H_2O which means that it is a compound of two parts hydrogen and one part oxygen.

If you drink rain water, or the fresh juices of fruits and vegetables, remember that all of this liquid has been distilled by nature.

If you drink rain water or snow water, there are no inorganic minerals in it. It is one hundred percent mineral-free.

If you drink fruit and vegetable juices, you are drinking distilled water, plus certain nutrients such as natural sugar, organic minerals, and vitamins.

But if you drink pure lake water, river water, well water, or spring water, you are drinking undistilled water, plus the inorganic minerals that the water has picked up.

Some of this water is known as hard-water, meaning that it has high concentrations of inorganic minerals.

Now, let me give you a short lesson in chemistry. There are two kinds of chemicals - inorganic and organic.

The inorganic chemicals are inert... which means that they cannot be absorbed into the living tissues of the body.

Our bodies are composed of 16 organic minerals, which must come from that which is living or has lived. When we eat an apple or any other fruit or vegetable, that substance is living. It has a certain length of life after it has been picked from the vine or tree. The same goes for animal foods, fish, milk, cheese, and eggs.

Organic minerals are vital in keeping us alive and healthy. If we were cast away on an uninhabited island where nothing was growing, we would starve to death. Because, even though the soil beneath our feet contains 16 inorganic minerals, our bodies could not absorb them. Only the living plant has the power to extract inorganic minerals from the earth. No human can extract nourishment out of inorganic minerals.

Many years ago I was on an expedition in China, and one part of the country was suffering from draught and famine. I saw with my own eyes poor, starving people heating earth and eating it, for want of food. They died horrible deaths, because they could not get one bit of nourishment from the inorganic minerals of the earth.

For years I have heard people say that certain waters were rich in all the minerals. What minerals are they talking about? Inorganic or organic? They are simply burdening their bodies with these inert minerals, which may cause the development of stones in the kidneys and gall bladder and acid crystals in the arteries, veins, and other parts of the body.

I was reared in a part of Virginia where the drinking water is called "hard water." It is heavily saturated with inorganic minerals, especially sodium, iron, and calcium. I saw many of my adult relations and friends die of kidney troubles. Nearly all of the people were prematurely-old, because the inorganic minerals would collect on the inner walls of the arteries and veins, causing them to die with hardening of the arteries. One of my uncles died at the great Johns Hopkins hospital in Baltimore, Maryland, when he was only 48 years of age. The doctors who performed the autopsy after death stated that his arteries were as hard as clay pipes, because they were so corroded with inorganic minerals.

Yet you will hear people say "Distilled water is dead water...a fish cannot live in it." Of course a fish cannot live in freshly-distilled water for any length of time, because he needs the vegetation that grows in rivers, lakes, and seas.

Let me put it another way... suppose you were on a big passenger ship going to Japan. Suppose the ship was wrecked and you and some other people were cast away in a lifeboat for days on the open sea. If the only water available was rain water, would you say "Rain water is distilled water, and because it is dead I will not drink it." Of course you would drink it and survive until you were rescued. You would be joining millions of people all over the world who drink rain water exclusively. Man evolved on drinking rain water. In Bermuda, the soil is so porous that water cannot be held in the soil, so people have special roofs to catch all rain water, draining it to a concrete reservoir under the house.

The great castle of the powerful emperor Tiberius on the Isle of Capri...who was world ruler at the time of Christ - has a remarkable reservoir to catch rain water, inside the castle walls. Today, 2000 years later, the people of Capri still go to this reservoir for water during a dry spell. I have seen this with my own eyes. If you visit the Isle of Capri, you, too, can see it today.

Years ago, when the late Douglas Fairbanks, Senior, and I were close friends, we roamed the South Sea Islands for several months, and during that trip, we came upon an island inhabited by beautiful, healthy Polynesians who never drank any water but distilled water, because the island was surrounded by the Pacific Ocean. This sea water was undrinkable because of the high salt content. Their island was based on porous coral which could not hold water...so they would only drink rain water, or the fresh, clear, clean water of the green coconut. I have never seen any finer specimens of men or women than these native South Sea Islanders. There were several doctors on the yacht who thoroughly examined the oldest people on these islands, and one heart doctor stated that he had never examined such well-preserved people in his life. You noted that I said only the most mature people were examined by our doctors...they were completely unaware of age because no such word existed in their language. They never celebrated birthdays, so they were gloriously ageless...not only in years but in body. These older men performed as well in the vigorous native dances as the younger men. They were beautiful specimens of manhood and womanhood, and they had lived their lengthy lives drinking only distilled water.

A few years ago I made an expedition to the far-off Atlas mountains of Morocco...here again I found vigorous people roaming the vast desert wastes, and the only water they drank was rain water.

Every liquid prescription that is compounded in any drug store in the world over is prepared with distilled water.

It is not true that distilled water leaches the organic minerals out of the body and it is not dead water. It is the purest water that man can drink!

Distilled water helps to dissolve the terrible, morbid, putrid, toxic poisons that collect in civilized men's bodies. It passes

through the kidneys without leaving inorganic pebbles and stones.
It is soft water. If you wash your hair in distilled water, you
will discover how soft it is. Note: No new water has been put
on the face of the earth since it was originally formed. Just as
the same energy is formed and re-formed, so the same water is
usable over and over again by the miracle of nature. Waters of
the earth are purified by distillation. The sun evaporates the
water...it is collected into clouds and the clouds become full and
then we have rain and dew...pure, perfectly clean water, one of
God's and Nature's great miracles. Who dares to say that God
and Nature supply man with dead water! Distilled water is the
purest water on the face of the earth and it is absolutely free of
all harmful inorganic substances.

Over 50 years ago, I predicted that some day man would need
clean, pure water so desperately that great government distill-
ing plants would be installed at the seas to convert the unlimited
supply of salt water into pure water for all purposes.

I have lived to see that prediction come true. At the great
American military base at Guantanamo Bay in Cuba, all the water
used for thousands of military personnel is clean, pure distilled
water.

In the American Navy, there are huge carriers with five thousand
Navy personnel aboard. These ships cannot carry enough land
water so they distill sea water for the men to drink - and bathin.

At my home in Hollywood, California, distilled water is delivered
in 5-gallon bottles for our household use, and I also have it at my
office. It can be purchased in almost every supermarket in the
nation. It is used in baby formulas and for many hundreds of
other purposes.

In thousands of homes, there are water softeners for household
uses, because hard water is not good for the hands, body or in
washing clothes. But please do not drink the water from water
softeners...and in my opinion it is not a healthful drinking water.
Try distilled water exclusively for a year and you will never
drink hard water again. Please never use hard water for a fast
...only distilled water.

★ ★ ★ ★ ★

Health is the most natural thing in the world.
It is natural to be healthy because we are a part
of nature - we are nature. Nature is trying
hard to keep us well, because she needs us in
her business.

- Elbert Hubbard

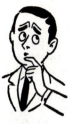

7

HOW LONG SHOULD ONE FAST?

For a person who has had no fasting experience, the longest fast should never be over ten days, unless he is under the strict supervision of some qualified person with years of successful fasting experience.

Fasting is, after all, a scientific method of purifying the body, and should be conducted scientifically. In my opinion, 60 to 70% of the so-called "healthy" people of today, and 85 to 95% of the seriously ill people would die from the effects of loosening the tremendous toxic poison they have stored in their bodies, if they tried a long fast, say of 21 to 35 days.

A long fast must be supervised by an expert, because he can better determine when a fast should be broken. Sometimes even the experts cannot tell how long a fast should last. When and how to break the fast is determined by watching carefully how conditions in the faster's body change during the fast. The expert watches to see how fast the kidneys are throwing off poisons. He examines the urine several times a day, and if too much toxic poison is being eliminated, causing a strain on the kidneys, the fast is broken at once.

So, even the greatest experts do not say to a person "You will now be put on a 30- or 40-day fast". I have often started people on a fast that I approximated would last 21 to 25 days. But, in the first six days, so many toxic poisons were released into the circulation, that I broke the fast at once. The faster was then given a natural diet, and in several weeks more fasting was attempted. But, it was always broken if there was too much elimination.

I have heard unqualified people say "the longer the fast, the greater the internal purification". This I definitely do not believe, because modern civilized man is the sickest animal on the face of the earth, none of God's other creatures have attempted to violate the laws of nutrition as much as man; no other creature on this earth eats with such utter lack of discretion as modern man!

I want it definitely understood that man cannot break a natural law. He breaks himself while attempting to break the natural law. Can man break the law of gravity? Can man jump off a 25-story building and live? Of course he cannot. This applies also to the nutritional laws of nature. Man has been brainwashed into eating the processed, devitalized, and dead food of civilization which has propelled him into such a pitiful, physical condition. Man is so gullible to the false propaganda that is passed out to him by the big "special interests" describing what healthy and long-lived people we are. Sickness is costly. Who spends more money for doctors, nurses, hospitals, surgery and drugs?

WE DO

Who spends more money in the pursuit of health than any other nation in the whole, wide world?

WE DO

Which nation has more "drives" to collect funds to fight the many diseases that plague our population?

WE DO

Who has more convalescent homes, clinics, and sanatoriums than any other country in the world?

WE DO

What nation spends the most money on magazines, newspaper, T.V., and radio advertising on "do-it-yourself", over-the-drug-counter medication?

WE DO

What nation takes the most aspirin and other so-called pain killers?

WE DO

We even have a special aspirin for children, because even they need pain-killers. In my opinion, aspirin in any form, or kind, buffered, plain, or mixed with other compounds is a potentially dangerous drug, and people who use too much are running serious risks.

Here again is another reason I do not believe in long fasts unless they are carefully supervised by an expert. The average person is not only filled with toxic poison from wrong food, air pollution, water pollution with chemicals, and salt...but they also have a residue of the many drugs they have consumed, that are stored deep in the organs of the body.

So, a long fast to cleanse one's body thoroughly sounds good in theory... but, in actual practice, emphatically "NO"!

In my fasting experience, I have achieved greater benefits from short fasts than I have by the long fasts, even though I have supervised many long fasts.

Starting with a 24- to 36-hour fast weekly, I find that the faster can really give himself a splendid internal housecleaning. With the no-breakfast plan except fruit (I do not call fresh fruit a full meal... it can be regarded as an nutritional refreshment). Along with a program of eating only whole natural foods, the person who really wishes to attain vitality supreme and agelessness, can prepare himself for a fast of from 3 to 4 days in several months.

After the weekly fast, and four to six fasts of from 3 to 4 days, for about four months, a person would be ready for a seven-day fast. By this time, large amounts of toxic waste have been removed from the body by the weekly fasts, the 3- and 4-day fasts, and the good, wholesome, natural diet.

With a background of 6 months of internal cleansing the seven-day fast will prove quite simple. This first seven-day fast will be a wonderful experience because the internal purification the faster receives will be tremendous!

In several more months, this person will be ready for a ten-day fast, and again, this will cause a super-cleansing of every cell in the body.

THE FASTER WILL GATHER GREAT EXPERIENCE

On this sensible, logical program of internal purification, you will be so imbued with the joys of a new life that fasting will become a necessary part of life itself. Day by day, while you watch the miracle of rejuvenation taking place in your body and mind, you will rejoice that you have been led to a program of right living that makes you a better person every day of your life.

HOW LONG SHOULD ONE FAST?

Most people spend the major part of their short lives destroying themselves, but we, who have found the light, have dedicated our lives to radiant living. It all comes down to the law of compensation... you get out of an effort just what you put into it! To me, any effort to achieve vitality supreme and ageless-ness is worth the effort. I have found what I want in life.

I know that money cannot buy health, long life, and agelessness. I know my true values.

Every day we read about wealthy men and women who are desperately ill...many of them dying long before they should. There is no wealth that can equal health and agelessness...that is the reason I often tell people I am the richest man on earth...I am a health multibillionaire! I have the greatest wealth a person can have...I have super-health 365 days of the year. I have a painless, tireless, and ageless body.

No one gave me my Health-Wealth...I earned it by living on a natural-health program...and by always staying as close to nature as possible in this poisoned world of today.

THE MORE OFTEN YOU FAST - THE LONGER YOU WILL BE ABLE TO FAST

I do not want to limit your fasting to ten days. But I do not advise fasting any longer than ten days until you have had, at the very least, six ten-day fasts spaced at three-month intervals. With that experience behind you, you could graduate to a fifteen-day fast. By then you have done a tremendous amount of internal house-cleaning. You know just what to expect from the fast. If you should attempt a 21- or 30-day fast you now know how to conduct the fast. You have had good experience behind you.

Personally, I feel that my weekly 24- to 36-hour fast and my 7- to 10-day fasts 4 times a year, is sufficient fasting for me. I eat only 12 meals a week, and sometimes less because I never eat unless I have a genuine hunger!

Again let me state emphatically that fasting is a science... Please do not force yourself into a long fast because you think the long fast is going to do wonders, except under the strict supervision of an expert. And even the expert may decide that you would benefit more from shorter fasts to first condition yourself to the longer fast.

Your 24- and 36-hour weekly fast...your 3- or 4-day fasts... your 7- to 10-day fasts will prepare you with the experience you will definitely need should you wish to try a longer fast later.

I personally don't believe in the longer fast unless it is really an emergency, and then it is imperative that it should be supervised by an expert. I have thousands of students around the world following the program I have prepared for you in this manuscript. They are delighted and satisfied with the marvelous results they have had!

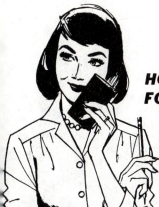

8

HOW LONG SHOULD ONE FAST FOR BEST BENEFITS?

I have found in my research on fasting that even the experts disagree on how long one should fast to get the very best results.

Many of the fasting resorts in England feel that the thirty-day fast is best. So, most people who go to an English fasting resort take the thirty-day fast. Under English supervision the faster is kept in bed most of the time, and is allowed to get up for only a few minutes at a time.

The German fasting resorts believe the ideal fast is twenty-one days. The French are in favor of not more than a fourteen day fast.

In our American fasting resorts most of the fasts are supervised for thirty days.

I have found that in foreign and American fasting resorts, the directors are dedicated men and women who have a thorough knowledge of fasting, and they have been highly successful with people who have various complicated physical problems.

Fasting is a great and wonderful science and there is much to learn about it.

I have been supervising fasts for over 70 years, and during this time, I have fasted faithfully every year with wonderful results.

It is my honest opinion that if anyone fasts over ten days, they should be under the supervision of an expert.

I believe that the average person can fast ten days without any complications. The ten-day fast results in a great amount of internal house-cleaning. I sincerely hope I am not putting any fear-thoughts in your mind about the great science of fasting. There are hundreds of people all over the world who supervise

their own fasts for 30 days or even more. In my travels around
the world giving health lectures, when I speak on fasting, I ask
my students how many of them have supervised their own fasts.
I found that I have many, many students who have fasted 30 days
or more, achieving great results.

But, I still feel that if a person is going to take a 30-day fast, he
should be under the supervision of an expert, who knows how to
control the fast. They are always ready to help you when the
toxic poisons are being eliminated more heavily. Many times
these experts may advise you to break the fast, because they
feel that you may have loosened enough toxic poisons for this
particular fast.

I BELIEVE IN SHORT FASTS WITH GOOD NUTRITION AND GOOD LIVING HABITS BETWEEN FASTS

I personally feel that the wheels of the Gods grind slowly, but
surely.

Here is my theory on the science of fasting. First, we are
dealing with human nature and there are many fears in each of
us. I believe that more people will experiment with the science
of fasting if they are short fasts. Many people are willing to try
a 24-hour fast or a 36-hour fast and when they find that they feel
better and look better, they will then attempt a three-day fast,
because they now have confidence. And the next thing you know,
they will fast from 7- to 10-days. And a 7- to 10-day fast is
highly successful. Many of my students who took several 10-day
fasts had such good results that they tried a 15-day fast. Some
even went on to 21 days and others tried the full 30-day fast,
under their own supervision.

But they first started with the 24-hour fast and graduated to the
longer fast. The more experience you gain, the stronger belief
you will have in fasting.

If you have never fasted before...start with one day a week on a
24-hour or 36-hour fast. I urge you to be the judge of the
wonder-working power of the fast.

Then you may graduate to the 3- to 4-day fast and, after that, to
a 7- to 10-day fast that will make you very proud of your will-
power. You can accomplish a great amount of internal cleansing
on short fasts, and remember it is accumulative...the more you
fast, the cleaner you become inside...and between fasts you are
living a good Health life.

★ ★ ★ ★ ★

Nothing transforms anyone as much as changing
from a negative to a positive attitude.

HERE IS MY PERSONAL FASTING PROGRAM AND
THE ONE I HIGHLY RECOMMEND TO MY STUDENTS

I know the great benefits I have received from fasting, and that
goes for my whole family.

Every week I take a 24-hour or a 36-hour fast.
This I never miss! In addition I fast from
seven to ten days, four times a year.

Over the many years that I have been following this schedule, I
have kept myself in a superior state of Health. I am a human
dynamo. I get more living out of one day than the average person gets out of five. I have an unlimited amount of energy for
work and play! I never get tired...sleepy - yes...but never do
I get that worn-out, exhausted feeling. I keep myself active
mentally, physically, and spiritually! I maintain a heavy lecture
schedule, and I travel all over the world...I write and have
many duties to perform. But I still have time for an enormous
amount of vigorous physical activity.

All of my play-time is spent with young men and women, except
for the older boys and girls who do not recognize calendar years
and who are young in body and mind, as I am. Otherwise I keep
far, far away from prematurely-old men and women, because
they are so negative. They have convinced themselves so often
that they are old and broken, and that is the reason they are
ready for the scrap heap! Many of them mentally died 30 or
more years ago and they are only walking around to save funeral
expenses.

I belong to hiking clubs, tennis clubs, beach clubs, mountain-
climbing clubs, dancing clubs...I am continually where the
action is. I love the new active dances...the twist...the watusi
...the mashed potato - any dance that gives me a chance to be
physically active, and mentally joyous.

For years I have been a student of the Hula and I love to swing
and sway to Hawaiian music. In fact, when I lecture in the
Hawaiian Islands I hold lively dancing parties at my home and
we have enormous fun doing the Hula.

When your body is cleansed by fasting and you are living a
natural Health life, you will discover that you feel wonderful all
the time. This is because Nature intended man to be a happy,
well-balanced person...free of fears, of frustrations, stresses
and strains. ★ ★ ★ ★ ★

The best service a book can render you is,
to impart truth, but to make you think it out for yourself.
—Elbert Hubbard

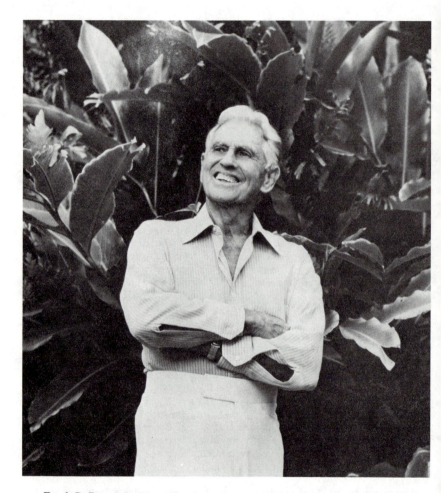

Paul C. Bragg in Hawaii, where he spends much of his time during the latter years of his vigorous, long life (almost a century). It is here that many Bragg health books are written. After a morning of swimming, and leading His "Long Life, Health and Happiness Club" (see page 100) in exercises, Paul often spends the rest of the day writing . . . to carry his message of healthful living to millions of students throughout the world.

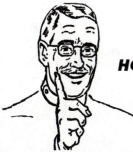

HOW TO BREAK A 24-HOUR FAST

9

HOW TO BREAK A 24-HOUR FAST

FOLLOW THE INSTRUCTIONS
CAREFULLY IN THIS CHAPTER

Your 24-hour fast can be from lunch to lunch, or from dinner to dinner, as long as you abstain from all solid foods, fruit, and this means also no fruit or vegetable juices! This is known as the absolute distilled water fast.

There is only one exception in the 24-hour fast. In each glass of distilled water, you may add one-third teaspoon of uncooked honey and one teaspoon of lemon juice. This acts as a mucus and toxic dissolver. It is not to help you "keep up your strength". It is to make the water more palatable and as I have said, to be used as a dissolver of mucus and toxic poisons, so they can be flushed out through the great natural sieve of the human body - the kidneys. The kidneys play a vital part in the one-day fast, the 36-hour fast, or the 7 to 10 day or longer fast. This is why it is important during any fast to drink copious amounts of distilled water.

I have told you how important it is to save the urine after a 24-hour fast and put it in a tightly sealed bottle on a shelf, and let it cool and settle for several weeks. You will see with your own eyes the poisons, such as mucus and toxins that have been flushed out of the body by the wonder-working kidneys.

THE MIRACLE ORGANS

Just think of it - each of the two kidneys in your body have a million efficient filters and when the body is fasting, the kidneys step up their work of detoxification. All of the vital force and nervous energy of the body is now working overtime because it is not being used up in the laborious task of mastication, digestion, metabolism, and elimination. You have no idea how powerful the Vital Force is in your body until you experience this great body renovation.

Again I would say that, as long as there is toxic waste in your circulation you may feel miserable during your fast, but as soon as the Vital Force flushes these poisons out through the kidneys, you will start to feel much better.

Many times during a fast, old drugs that have been buried in your system for years are loosened up and flushed out of the body. Let me

63

tell you of one of my greatest experiences when I first started fasting. Now let's go back to my early childhood diet...I was born and reared in Virginia, and I was fed a typical heavy, greasy, starchy, fatty, and sugary diet. My body was so filled with acid as a child that I had every known childhood disease; mumps, measles, whooping cough - you name them and I had them. Along with these childhood miseries, I was given large amounts of a drug known as "calomel" and this drug was filled with quicksilver.

SWISS DOCTOR MY SAVIOR

After I was restored to a good state of health at Dr. August Rollier's Sanitarium in Leysen, Switzerland, I started my regular fasting program...which I am proud to say I have continued through all these wonderful years since then! I fasted one 24-hour period weekly and four times a year at three-month intervals, I fasted from 7 to 10 days, always on a strict distilled-water fast. After I had been on this program for 5 years, I went on a 10-day fast and a miracle happened to me. I was at my families old homestead in Virginia, and on about the seventh day of the ten-day fast, I was out in a canoe on the river leisurely enjoying the sunshine and fresh air, when suddenly, without warning, I doubled up with stomach cramps and I thought I would never be able to stand the pain. With great effort I got ashore and then it happened. I had a terrific bowel evacuation, and at the end of this evacuation, I felt a heavy cool sensation in my rectum and out passed a third of a cup of the quicksilver from the Calomel that I had taken during my childhood. That experience marked a new day in my entire physical structure. From that day on, I knew what superior health meant! My Vital Power had increased so greatly with this program of eating natural, living foods, fasting, and using all of the natural forces of Nature, such as fresh air, sunshine, exercise and bathing, that every cell of my body seemed to rejoice with a new Power of Vitality!

In my opinion, I believe that over the years I have eliminated the residue of many of the drugs that were given to me for childhood miseries.

KEEP YOUR MORALE HIGH

I want you to understand that even when you take the one day fast, you are cleansing and purifying your whole body. The very thought that you are building a painless, tireless, ageless body should be an incentive to keep your morale high during your fast. Don't allow self-pity, or any negative thoughts, to get in your mind during your fast. Repeat these powerful affirmations all during the day you are fasting.

1. I have this day put my body in the hands of God and Nature. I have turned to the highest power for internal purification and rejuvenation.

2. Every minute that I am fasting, I am flushing dangerous poisons out of my wonderful body that could do great damage. Every hour that I am fasting, I am happier and happier.

3. Hour by hour my body is purifying itself.

4. In fasting, I am using the same method for physical, mental and spiritual purification that the greatest spiritual leaders have used throughout the ages.

5. I am in complete control of my body during this fast. No false hunger habit-pains are going to make me stop fasting. I will carry my fast through to a successful conclusion, because I have absolute faith in God and Nature!

Just remember you must direct instructions to the cells of your body with your subconscious mind. Whatever thought you send to your body is going to be carried out by your cells. That is the reason I urge you to never discuss your fasting program with relatives, your friends, or your acquaintances! All you will get is a negative reaction. Fasting is a personal matter, so keep it that way. When the toxins are passing out of your body and your circulation, and you feel uncomfortable, just say to yourself, "This will also pass". Be strong-minded when you fast, by thinking of the wonderful results you are going to achieve by purification...rejoice that you have been led to this great natural miracle.

At the end of the 24-hour fast, the very first food that reaches your taste buds, should be a raw variety vegetable salad with a base of grated carrots and grated cabbage. (Use either juice of lemon or orange over salad as dressing.) This will act as a broom in the 30 feet of intestines. It will give the muscles along the gastrointestinal tract something to work with. You can follow this salad with one or two cooked vegetables. They should be 5-percent vegetables, such as fresh stewed tomatoes. Stewed tomatoes are not acid-forming, except when you prepare them with refined, devitalized white sugar or hunks of refined, chemicalized white bread. You may have a serving of any kind of greens, such as spinach, kale, or chard; you may have squash, cooked celery, or string beans.

Remember, you should never break a fast with animal products such as meat, milk, cheese, butter, fish; nuts, or seeds. Your first meal must be composed of a raw salad and 5-percent vegetables. After a 24-hour or a 36-hour fast, wait until the 2nd

meal before you eat any of the above products that I have
mentioned.

HOW TO CONDUCT A 3-DAY, 7-DAY
AND A 10-DAY FAST

A fast of 3 days or more should be conducted under ideal conditions. You should be able to rest any time you feel the poisons
passing out of your body. During this time you might feel most
uncomfortable, and you should be able to go to your bed and relax there in quiet until the poisons have passed out of the body.
You should not read, view television, listen to the radio, or have
company of any kind. You should retire to your bedroom and
remain absolutely in seclusion. This period of discomfort will
leave as soon as the loosened poisons have passed out of your
system through the kidneys.

Again I repeat that, during the longer fast you should not tell
anyone what you are doing, because they will project innumer-
able negative thoughts to you at a time when you must keep only
positive thoughts of the miracle that is happening in your body
during your fast.

My fasting is such a personal thing that many years ago in
California, I went into the Santa Monica Mountains and found a
tract of land in the wilderness of the Topanga Canyon. There I
built a small cabin and used it for a retreat. In that seclusion I
often conduct my fasts. If it is possible for you to get away to
some secluded place and do your fast in fresh air and solitude,
you will have better results!

There are also some very fine fasting institutions in our country
where all the conditions are perfect for a fast...many of my
good students who fast regularly tell me that they use their vacation period as a period of fasting and purification. They will go
to some beautiful spot and rent a room and there they will take
their fast in seclusion. I am not saying that it is necessary to
go away to fast because your home is your castle and you are
more likely to be at peace there. My family are all fasters, and
when anyone of us is fasting, we have great consideration for
each other. We have an agreement not to ask each other how we
feel during the fast. Fasting is so personal that no one can do
anything for you during the fast, so the best thing is not to discuss it with anyone, not even with one who is in sympathy with
your action. WHEN YOU ARE ON A FAST FROM 3 TO 10 DAYS
OR MORE, YOU ARE REALLY ON NATURE'S OPERATING
TABLE. Nature is ridding you of the waste, mucus, toxins, and
other foreign substances in your body.

★ ★ ★ ★ ★

*Now I see the secret of the making of the best persons, it is to grow in the open air, and eat
and sleep with the earth.*
—Walt Whitman

66

So again let me reiterate, any fast of 3 days or more should be conducted under the most ideal conditions.

Bed rest is vitally important because all your vital power must be used for detoxication and internal cleansing. During your fast, if you feel that you want to take a little walk in the fresh air, or you would like to take a sun-bath, only do it if you feel strong. Don't take a long sun-bath because often a long sun-bath is enervating, and exercise also lessens the vitality. Don't do anything that would deplete your energy! During the years that I had my fasting resort, I told my students, who were fasting, that the best results of a 3- to 10-day fast, came when the students had plenty of bed rest. If the faster can sleep, the more he sleeps during the fast, the better. If there are periods when it is impossible to sleep, simply relax, let yourself go. It is good to just cut yourself off from the world once in a while. Don't think of your business problems or your home, empty your mind of everything, and let yourself go completely.

DON'T WORRY ABOUT YOUR BOWELS MOVING DURING THE FAST

One of the greatest worries most fasters have during a fast of from 3 to 10 days is that the bowels may stop moving. Let me emphasize, don't worry about bowel movement during a fast! This will adjust itself shortly after the fast is broken. I do not believe in laxatives or enemas during the fast, so forget all about bowel movements and think about the wonderful purification that your body is experiencing. I don't believe in an enema any time ... I don't believe in forcing nature and the use of the enema, in my opinion, is most unnatural. This includes taking any kind of laxative before or during the fast. The bowel has its own sanitary and antiseptic machiners, and the residue that was in your bowel at the beginning of your fast will be neutralized until the fast is over. Nature's plumbing system is perfect if you will allow it to work naturally. When the fast is over and you eat meals that are well-balanced in bulk, moisture and lubrication, your bowels will move more naturally than they ever did, because you are going to eat 50 percent of your foods in their raw natural state in the form of salads and fruits.

You are going to eat plenty of light, leafy, 5-percent vegetables. You are not going to eat meat and fish over three times a week. The balance of your protein needs will be met by nuts, seeds and vegetables. If you eat whole grain breads of any kind, you will toast them and let them cool (this is known as Melba Toast). Any bread you eat should always be dextrinized; that is, it should be toasted until the starch is converted into what we call "blood sugar". Melba toast should be so well toasted that you can take it in your hand and make a powder out of it. After the fast you are going to use raw wheat germ, the most important part of wheat. This is a food that furnishes the body with bulk, moisture, and lubrication.

Instructions on selecting a superior diet for good nutrition appears further on in this book.

NORMAL COLON AND SICK COLONS

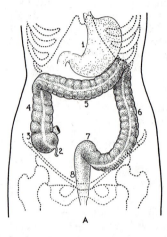

A

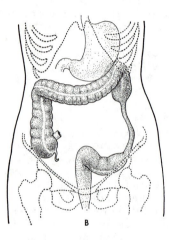

B

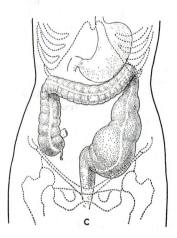

C

A, The normal large bowel or colon in the proper position in relation to other structures: 1, stomach; 2, appendix; 3, cecum; 4, ascending colon; 5, transverse colon; 6, descending colon; 7, sigmoid flexure; 8, rectum.
B, The colon in spastic constipation.
C, The colon in atonic constipation.
D, Ptosis, or sagging, of the transverse colon, accompanied by displacement of the stomach.

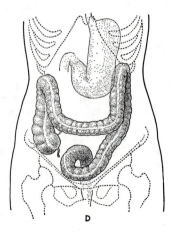

D

10

I FAST 7 TO 10 DAYS FOUR TIMES A YEAR

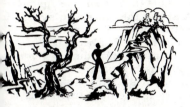

The Trail To Perfect Health

I am very sincere about my fasting program. I know what it has done for me, for the members of my family, my friends, and thousands of my health-conscious students all over the world.

So my program calls for 4 fasts a year, along with a weekly 24-hour or 36-hour fast.

At the beginning of each year, I mark the days that I am going to fast from 7 to 10 days. Now you may wonder why I say 7 to 10 days. The reason I sometimes fast only 7 days is because I feel that in that time I have accomplished the necessary house-cleaning of my body.

I have fasted for so many years that I am perceptive to what a fast is doing for me. An inner voice seems to tell me when to break the fast. So, my calendar calls for a fast in the first part of January. As I say, sometimes this fast lasts 7 days; it may run 8 days; it may run 9 days; and it may extend the full 10 days.

I then mark on my calendar a fast for the early spring. My spring fast always runs 10 days, because that is when I want to truly clean house after a long winter. In my lecture work, I am often forced to talk in over steamheated halls and auditoriums. I am sorry to say that most humans cannot take cold weather, nor can they stand a fresh, healthily ventilated hall. So I must forget my feelings and lecture in these overheated halls to the hothouse plants of civilization that people have become.

★ ★ ★ ★ ★

"God gave his creatures light and air
and water open to the skies;
Man locks him in a stifling lair
and wonders why his brother dies."

- Oliver Wendell Holmes

FASTING BUILDS A NATURAL THERMOSTAT
INTO THE BODY

I feel that fasting so purifies the body, so exhilarates the functions of the body by internal purity, that the thermostatic system of the body works with absolute efficiency. For instance,
I can leave my desert home near Palm Springs, California, in
January when the thermometer averages in the 80's during the
day and the nights in the 60's. I can board an airplane to mid-
western cities, such as Duluth or Minneapolis, Minnesota, or
to a Canadian City such as Toronto where the temperature will
be as low as 10 to 30 degrees below zero. Because of fasting
and natural living, my body will adjust easily to this bitter cold
weather. In fact, I can take the most frigid weather better than
the inhabitants who are already acclimated to their climate.

This ability to adjust to climate is only one of the many marvelous things that happen to the body when you fast, giving it a
chance to flush out the toxic poisons and build Vital Power.

But, as I have stated, when I go to the cities that are locked in
freezing weather, I find that their halls and auditoriums are
overheated. There is so little oxygen in the air, that naturally
my body will absorb some of the carbon dioxide that people
expel from their lungs through the breathing process. That is
where my spring fasting becomes valuable. I want to flush out
of my body, with a 10-day fast, these accumulated toxic poisons
and the other poisons that are found in artificially-heated rooms.
So my fast in the springtime is always 10 days.

Then when summer rolls around, I take a 7-day fast in the latter
part of July or August. This is the easiest of all my fasts,
because I have been eating large amounts of luscious, fresh
fruit and garden-fresh, organically-grown vegetables. I believe
I enjoy my summer fast more than any other. In fact, the fast
is so easy that I never stop either heavy physical or mental
activities.

My autumn fast can be anywhere in late October or during
November, and it extends from 7 to 10 days.

As I told you, fasting has an accumulative effect. Since I fast
approximately 75 days a year, just think of the physiological
rest I give my digestive organs. This includes the liver, gall
bladder, and all the faithful organs within my body that are
manufacturing hormones. The physiological rest that I give
my pancreas allows it to produce ample insulin and that also
goes for the stomach where so many digestive juices are needed
to handle daily food. You will find that after a fast, you will
have more saliva in your mouth. You will find that your mouth

will taste sweeter, that your breath will be clean, and, strange as it may seem to you, the more you fast, the less body odor you will have.

NATURE INTENDED THE BODY AND BREATH TO BE SWEET AND FREE FROM ODOR

Several years ago, I supervised a fasting program for a student who came to California from New York. His problem was a terrifically bad body odor that exuded from every part of his body, particularly from under the arms, in the palm of his hands, and his feet. The odor can only be described as putrid. It wasn't that the man didn't take baths, because he told me that he had taken as many as 3 and 4 hot, soapy baths daily and would use all kinds of deodorants or anti-perspirants, but all to no avail for that horrible odor persisted. He was becoming a nervous wreck, because he felt like a social outcast. He not only had a bad body odor, but he had such heavy halitosis that I believe his breath would kill a mule. He used gargles, lozenges, and chewed heavily flavored chewing gum, but still that rancid breath persisted.

In questioning this man before the fast, I found that he had been enervated by overwork, marital difficulties, and heavy financial responsibilities. When you enervate yourself, when you over-expend your nervous energy and exhaust your vital power, then the organs of elimination cannot do their job effectively and efficiently. This man was plainly suffering from nerve exhaustion; his eating habits were unhealthy; his working day was so busy that he would gobble a sandwich and wash it down with coffee. He simply did not take the time to select a well-balanced and nourishing diet. His elimination thus functioned out of normal rhythm.

I told him that it had taken him years to get into this decaying condition and that fasting and a program of natural living would take time to accomplish its mission, but he was an intelligent and logical-thinking man and he cooperated with me as supervisor of his program, and gave me his undivided cooperation. I started him on a 36-hour fast, and between the fasts, I gradually added more raw fruit and vegetables to his heavily concentrated diet of refined carbohydrates and meats. I believe there must be a transition period between changing from a perverted diet to a natural diet. You cannot force the human body to change quickly. You must take things slowly. Instead of eating meat 3 times a day, he now ate meat only once a day. He had been a great eater of white bread, so I substituted 100-percent whole grain bread, Melba toasted. Then I gave him a 7-day fast. The first 3 days was rough, because he was now eliminating accumulated toxic poisons. He vomited off and on during the first 4 days, and on the 5th day he broke out in a rash. The odor that came from his body and his breath was absolutely unbearable. I almost needed a gas mask to get within 4 feet of him. I took a specimen of his urine every morning, the first urine of the day. I sealed it tightly, dated it, and let it sit on a shelf to settle and cool. It was absolutely unbelievable how, after a few weeks, such dark, cloudy urine could possibly come out of a human.

I am well acquainted with the odor of putrid urine, because I am a Physical Therapist, licensed by the State Board of Medical Examiners of the State of California, and in my long years as a Physical Therapist, working under many famous medical doctors, I spent a great deal of time in hospitals. I have smelt urine that came from sick people where the stench was unbearably sickening. In fact I have seen nurses and doctors who vomited when they smelt the urine coming from these dangerously sick people.

After the fast, I eliminated more of the civilized foods, added more raw fruits and vegetables, and after several more weeks, I gave my student a 10-day fast. This was a much easier fast for him, but he still eliminated heavy amounts of toxic matter. This is called "latent poison", and has concentrated in the cells of the body. It takes a long program of fasting and alkaline-feeding to dislodge this stored, deadly material. For instance, at my clubs or in my active social life, people will say to me, "Well, Mr. Bragg, with all due respect to your philosophy of living, I am a perfectly healthy person, I eat what agrees with me, I drink all the coffee I want, and I eat what any normal person eats." Then they proceed to tell me how strong they are, but I know better. I know that the poison is storing up in their tissues and I know that some day it will break loose, and they will become deathly ill as this healing crisis takes place. That is what sickness is — Nature trying to purify the body from an overload of toxic poison.

Now I am the first to admit that, through heredity, many people inherit constitutions of steel. They can laugh and flaunt every law of God and Nature and seem to get away with it, but the day of restitution always arrives ... the day when Nature starts a purification by some form of elimination. Believe me, I have seen these so-called, naturally-healthy people who could eat anything, drink anything, smoke, lose sleep, work 18 hours or more a day, crumble, and be carried off to the hospital. I have seen them writhe in pain, in such intense suffering that tears would well in my eyes from their extreme torture, and I am sorry to say, I have seen many of these powerful people go to an early grave.

★ ★ ★ ★ ★

A prudent man will think more important what faith has conceded to him than what it has denied.

So I knew that my student had to be handled very carefully. So it pleased me that he kept up his program persistently and faithfully. It took almost a year of fasting and natural living to defeat his annoying enemies. Today that man has a sweet, clean breath. There is no longer any putrid odor exuding from the pores of his body. He is an entirely different man. He not only defeated the enemies within his body, but he knocked off 20 years in his looks. He is now a handsome man, youthful-looking, vigorous-looking, with lots of personal magnetism; he is a man who is more relaxed because he has a tranquil mind. So it must be very obvious to you why I use a preventive method of living. Most people wait until something happens before they act, but I believe that an ounce of prevention is far better than a pound of cure.

Those of you who are reading this book should not wait until Nature shocks you into detoxication. Isn't it far more logical and sensible to give your body a physiological rest every week for 24 to 36 hours? Isn't it good sound reasoning to you to take a 7- to 10-day fast from time to time and give your body a chance to purify itself? Give your body a chance to get rid of the accumulative poisons. In our modern, complex civilization, we are absolutely bound to pick up poisons.

I have explained to you very thoroughly in this book that we live in a poisonous world, and that our only salvation is to go on a program of detoxification and internal purification. It can mean a whole new life for you! It can mean a life of happiness, because when you are healthy you are happy.

★★★★★★★★

Jesus proceeded to divide all actions into three major categories. These were: doing good to others —almsgiving), intimate relationship to God (prayer), and personal discipline (fasting is used as illustrative of the larger area of self-control). Jesus taught that life in His Kingdom required the right balance among these areas of involvement.

The Lord Jesus gave us clear directions to obey concerning almsgiving, prayer and fasting. Our obedience will bring us into a walk of balance.

But as for me, when they were sick, my clothing was sackcloth; I afflicted myself with fasting, and I prayed with head bowed on my breast.

--Psalms 35:13 AMPLIFIED

Morning Resolve

I will this day live a simple, sincere and serene life, repelling promptly every thought of impurity, discontent, anxiety, discouragement and self-seeking. I will cultivate cheerfulness, happiness, charity and the love of brotherhood; exercising economy in expenditure, generosity in giving, carefulness in conversation and diligence in appointed service. I pledge fidelity to every trust and a childlike faith in God, in particular, I will be faithful in those habits of prayer, study, work, physical exercise, deep breathing and good posture. I shall fast one 24 hour period each week, eat only natural foods and get sufficient sleep each night. I will make every effort to improve myself physically, mentally and spiritually every day.

Morning prayer used by Paul C. Bragg and Patricia Bragg

In the Beginning . . .

To find out what really happened when the earth was created, engineers spent weeks gathering information, checking and rechecking it, and feeding it into the computer. The great moment came: all was complete, everybody gathered around, a button was pressed, the great computer spun into action, relays opened and closed, lights flashed and bells rang, and finally a typed message emerged: "See Genesis 1:1." — The Anglican Digest

★★★★★★

"Give us, Lord, a bit of sun,
A bit of work and a bit of fun.
Give us, in all struggle and sputter,
Our daily whole grain bread and a bit of nut butter.
Give us health, our keep to make
And a bit to spare for others' sake.
Give us, too, a bit of song
And a tale and a book, to help us along.
Give us, Lord, a chance to be
Our goodly best for ourselves and others
'Til all men learn to live as brothers."

– An Old English Prayer

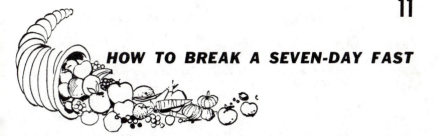

11

HOW TO BREAK A SEVEN-DAY FAST

Remember that when you have been on a 7-day fast, your
stomach and the 30 feet of intestinal tract have contracted,
and when you are ready to break the fast, it should be done
as follows:

Around 5 o'clock of the 7th day of the fast, peel 4 or 5 medium-
sized tomatoes, cut them up, bring them to a boil and then
turn off the heat, and when they are cool enough to eat, have
as many as you desire. On the morining of the 8th day, you are
to have a salad of grated carrots and grated cabbage, with half
an orange squeezed over it. After your salad, you may have a
bowl of steamed greens and peeled tomatoes (spinach, Swiss
chard, or mustard greens). Bring the greens to a boil, then
turn off the heat. With your greens, you may eat 2 slices of
100-percent whole-wheat bread which has been toasted until it
is thoroughly dry — this is called "Melba toast". After it has
cooled, the toast should be so dry that it would powder if you
squeezed it in the palm of your hand. As I have stated, this
first food should be in the morning. During the day you may
have all the distilled water you wish to drink.

For dinner you may have a salad of grated carrots, chopped
celery and cabbage, with orange juice for dressing. This will
be followed by 2 cooked vegetables ... one such as spinach,
kale, chard, or mustard greens, and one such as string beans,
carrots, steamed celery, okra, or squash. You may have 2
pieces of whole-grain "Melba toast". These meals are not to
contain oils of any kind.

On the morning of the 9th day, you may have a dish of any kind
of fresh fruit, such as banana, pineapple, orange, sliced grapefruit, or sliced apples. You may sprinkle this with 2 table-
spoonsful of raw wheat germ, and sweeten it with honey, but not
over one tablespoonful. At noon you may have a salad of grated
carrots, cabbage, and celery, with one cooked vegetable and one
slice of "Melba toast". At dinner you may have a salad dish of
lettuce, watercress, parsley and tomatoes, and 2 cooked
vegetables. Beginning the 10th day, you may use the menus
given on page 184 of this book.

HOW TO BREAK A TEN-DAY FAST

There is little difference between the 7- and the 10-day fast.
On the 10th day around 5 o'clock you will have stewed ,
tomatoes; from then you will follow the same schedule as
given in the 7-day fast.

IMPORTANT

Do not eat any more than you desire. Remember that you have
been without food for 7 to 10 days and, by this time, you have
lost the craving for food. Because you eat is no sign that you
are going to immediately feel a surge of energy. It takes time
for the body to adjust from a detoxicating program to an eating
program.

AGAIN — DO NOT WORRY ABOUT BOWEL EVACUATION

It may take the body a day or two to adjust to eating again, so
don't be concerned if your bowels are sluggish. In many
instances, some people will have a bowel evacuation shortly
after eating the first meal after the fast, but elimination is
different for each person, so we cannot set a standard when the
bowels will move regularly again. I urge you to be patient with
Nature, and don't try to force the bowels to move. Nature has
given the bowels their own sanitation and antiseptic system,
and this system will cause a natural movement eventually. You
are eating foods that stimulate the peristaltic or wormlike
motion of the bowels. When they do begin evacuation, if you
follow instructions and continue the menus on correct eating,
you will establish a regular and healthful system of elimination.

THE IDEAL ELIMINATION PROGRAM

In my own life, by living on a diet which is rich in bulk, moisture, and lubrication, I have established the following eliminative habits. I have a bowl elimination shortly after arising.
I encourage this by a few twisting movements of my body which
give me a full and complete elimination. As I told you, I do
not eat breakfast because I believe the non-breakfast plan is
more healthful. Several hours after arising, I eat a dish of
fresh fruit ... sliced pineapple, bananas, and oranges, or a
dish of organically-grown, unsulphured, cooked apricots. I
may have a dish of prunes. An hour or so later I have my first
meal of the day, usually a raw vegetable combination salad
with a base of grated carrots, cabbage and celery. To this, I
often add avocado, because I think the avocado mixed with the
cabbage, carrots, and celery is an excellent lubricant and
stimulant to the entire gastrointestinal tract. I make it a hard

and fast rule, to always eat my salad first. I do this for several reasons. First, I think we must educate our 260 taste buds to accept only natural foods, therefore when you have raw foods, either a raw vegetable salad or a fruit salad to start the meal, you educate the taste buds to demand clean, live foods.

Most people start a meal with a broth or soup, sandwiches, or bread. This is wrong, in my opinion. To make the taste buds keen, sharp, and alive, the raw food at the beginning of the meal starts the digestive juices flowing, because raw foods are rich in natural enzymes. All this contributes to good nutrition ... so I urge you to always eat something raw at the beginning of each meal, and you will find over the years that your taste buds will begin to reject any kind of devitalized and demineralized food that you may be tempted to eat. As you educate the 260 taste buds to enjoy raw foods, you will find that you can and should increase the amount of raw foods you eat to 60 percent of your total intake of food.

Just remember that the raw foods are the live, vital foods ... they are as Nature prepared them — they are whole foods, natural foods, live foods, vibrating with enzymes and solar energy.

Most people want food that stimulates them ... they want cooked foods that have been robbed of their vital elements.

I am not influencing you to eat a 100-percent raw food diet, because I don't think civilized man can live as his ancestors of 5 or 6 thousand years ago lived. That is why I believe that the ideal diet is made up of 3/5 of raw fruits and vegetables, and 1/5 protein. This protein can be in the form of meat, fish, eggs, natural cheese, or it can be in a vegetarian form, such as nuts, nut-butters, seeds, or seed meal, such as sunflower seeds, sesame seeds, or pumpkin seeds. Brewer's yeast and wheat germ also form an important part of your protein. The last fifth is divided into three. One-third of one-fifth are natural starches, such as whole-grains, in the form of bread or cereals, brown rice, dried legumes, such as lentils, all kinds of dried beans, garbanzos, dried lima beans, and dried lentils. The next one-third of the one-fifth is devoted to natural sugars, found in sun-dried fruits such as dates, figs, raisins, honey, maple syrup, unsulphured molasses, and black-strap molasses. The last one-third of the one-fifth of food is devoted to natural unsaturated oils, such as safflower oil, soya oil, olive oil, walnut oil, and any unsaturated natural oil.

The natural starches, sugars, and fats are highly concentrated foods, so they are within the smaller quantities.

VEGETARIANISM — MEAT-EATING

Over the 50 years or more that I have been a Nutritionist, the controversy of "Vegetarianism vs. Meat-eating" has raged furiously. Both sides present the most scientific reasons for their side of the story. I am not going to try to persuade you to be either a vegetarian or a meat-eater. There are hundreds of books written on both of these subjects. In my own life, I try to eliminate the word "NEVER" when it comes to food.

Over the years of following a program of fasting, and with a diet containing an abundance of raw fruit and raw vegetables, my body has become so keen that it practically tells me what to eat at every meal. Over the years on this diet, my body has lost the desire for meat and fish, and my diet is composed of raw fruits and vegetables, cooked fruit, and cooked vegetables with nuts, nut-butters, seeds, raw wheat germ, Brewer's yeast, and legumes.

This is what my body seems to thrive on, but as I said, I don't like the word "NEVER," because there are times when my body tells me to eat a piece of meat or a piece of fish, or to have some natural cheese or a few fertile eggs. In other words, my body has developed an instinct for the selection of foods. Sometimes I go 4 or 5 years without tasting either meat or fish, then my body will telegraph that I need a piece of meat or fish, and I eat it. This inner voice has helped me enormously.

Basically, I have been a vegetarian by nature all my life. I was reared on a large farm in Virginia where hundreds of hogs and cattle were slaughtered ... so killing has always been repulsive to me. I have never been a hunter or a fisherman, because I do not like to take another life. I have made 13 expeditions to primitive lands, and I have found many robust, healthy people living on a vegetarian diet. On the other hand, I have found people in primitive places who enjoyed higher health and yet included animal products in their diets. I roamed the South Seas for over a year at one time and in those far flung islands, I found supermen and women and they not only lived on an abundance of fresh fruit and vegetables, but they included fish, fowl, and some meat in their diet.

So you see, I have tried to be as fair as I could about this question of Vegetarianism vs. Meat-eating. I feel that as we cleanse and purify the body, we develop a keen sense of selection.

★ ★ ★ ★ ★ ★

"A temperate diet arms the body against all external accidents, So that they are not so easily hurt by the heat, cold or labor."

- Benjamin Franklin

SEVEN OF MY BELOVED TEACHERS

One of the greatest teachers and physicians in the science of body purification and nutrition was Dr. John Tilden, M.D., of Denver. This great scientist goes down in history as one of the finest physicians. His program included fasting and an abundance of fruits, vegetables, and animal products. He lived into his 90's and was an active physician until the day he died.

On the other hand, one of the finest doctors who specialized in nutrition was the famed Dr. John Harvey Kellogg, M.D., for 60 years the director of the famous Battle Creek Sanitarium in Battle Creek, Michigan. Dr. Kellogg specialized in a vegetarian diet and people from all over the world were restored to radiant health with a vegetarian diet. I had the privilege of studying under Dr. Kellogg and I felt it was one of the outstanding experiences of my life.

At the turn of the century, I was associated with Bernarr Macfadden, the father and founder of the Physical Culture Movement. Mr. Macfadden tried vegetarianism for a time, but finally went back to the mixed diet, which included meat and fish. He was another man who lived to be nearly 88 years of age and who believed in the mixed diet.

Over my many years in the nutritional field, I have met many famous men and women who restored hundreds of people to health again through the natural system of dietetics. In the early twenties, I had the privilege of working with Dr. St. Louis Estes, D.D.S., who was a pioneer and strict believer in a raw food diet. I saw many broken, weak, sick people restored to health by his raw food diet.

Dr. Benedict Lust, M.D., was the Father and Founder of Naturopathy in America. He established in New York a great school of Naturopathy and graduated hundreds of Nature Doctors who taught his teachings around the world.

Dr. Henry Lindlahr, M.D., was a Famous Drugless Physician who pioneered for the return to Natural Methods in the modern treatment and prevention of disease.

Professor Arnold Ehret, was one of the greatest food scientists in the world, in my opinion. He was the discoverer and creator of "THE MUCUSLESS DIET HEALING SYSTEM", which was strictly a vegetarian diet. I know many of Professor Ehret's students today who are in their eighties and nineties and who are enjoying vigorous, robust health by following his plan.

I could name many other food scientists with whom I have come in contact, and studied with, who practice either the mixed diet, the vegetarian diet, or the raw food diet, but they all had one thing in common, and that is that they eliminated all of the so-called, "processed and refined foods" of our civilization. Here is a list of foods that all of these great men of nutritional science believed should be eliminated from the diet:

FOODS TO AVOID

- Refined sugar or refined sugar products such as - jams - jellies - preserves - marmalades - ice cream - sherberts - Jello - cake - candy - cookies - chewing gum - soft drinks - pies - pastries - tapioca puddings - sugared fruit juices - fruits canned in syrup

- Catsup - mustard - Worchestershire sauce - pickles - green olives

- Salted foods, such as potato chips - salted nuts - pretzels - salted crackers, and sauerkraut

- White rice and pearled barley

- Commercial dry cereals such as corn flakes and other cereals.

- Fried foods

- Saturated fats and hydrogenated oils ... (enemies of your heart)

- Food which contains cottonseed oil. When a product is labeled vegetable oil ... find out what kind it is before you use it.

- Oleo and margarines ... (saturated fats and hydrogenated oils)

- Peanut butter that contains hydrogenated oils

- Coffee - decaffeined coffee - tea and alcoholic beverages

- Tobacco

- Fresh pork and pork products

- Smoked fish of any kind

- Smoked meats, such as ham - bacon and sausage

FOODS TO AVOID

- Lunch meats, such as hot dogs - salami - bologna - corned beef - pastrami, and any meats containing sodium nitrate or nitrite

- Dried fruits which contain sulphur dioxide ... (preservative)

- Do not eat chickens that have been injected with stilbestrol, or fed with chicken feed that contains any drugs

- Canned soups (read labels ... look for sugar - starch - white or wheat flour, and preservatives)

- Food that contains benzoate of soda, cream of tartar ... (preservatives)

- White flour products such as white bread - wheat-white bread - rye bread that has wheat-white flour in it - dumplings - biscuits - buns - gravy - noodles - pancakes - waffles - soda crackers - macaroni - - spaghetti - pizza pie - ravioli - sago - pies - pastries - cakes - cookies - prepared and commercial puddings - and ready-mix bakery products

- Bleached and unbleached flour products

- Day-old vegetables - pre-mixed salads - and warmed-over potatoes

- Self drugging - no aspirin, buffered aspirin, antihistamines, milk of magnesia, sleeping pills, tranquilizers, pain killers, strong cathartics, or fizzing bromides. You are not qualified to prescribe drugs for yourself (results can be serious).

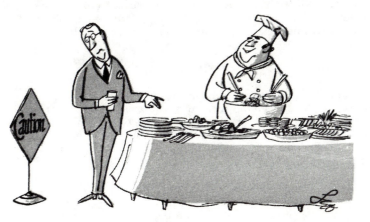

12

I DO NOT BELIEVE IN THE ENEMA DURING THE FAST

I have read many books on fasting and a majority of them recommend that, during the fast, a daily enema should be taken. I want it emphatically understood that I do not believe in the enema during fasting or any other time except in the direst emergency. When the bowel absolutely refuses to evacuate, or in times of illness, it is to be regarded only as a "crutch."

In comparing the enema to a powerful laxative, I would say that the enema is superior to the drug laxative, but it also has its own faults. Continued over a long period of time, it will set up irritation and wash out important internal and mucous membrane secretions and evacuate the bacteria necessary for good bowel function. It washes away the "goodies" in the form of beneficial bacteria; Nature, abhorring a vacuum, makes the entrance of the "Bad Bacteria" very easy — hence, infection.

During a fast you are having a physiological rest! Since no food is being eaten, the wave-like motion called "peristalsis" stops. The whole eliminative system is having a complete rest during the fast, and you must not disturb it during the rest period. The body has its own sanitation and antiseptic system within the bowel, so in many instances there will be no defecation of the bowels during a fast. Don't worry about it, and don't use an enema or a laxative. Allow the bowel to rest, this is why you are fasting. The whole idea is to give the great eliminative system of your body a complete rest.

From time to time, during a fast, there may be some bowel elimination. But if there is none, you are not going to be poisoned. When you start eating natural foods after the fast, the bowel elimination will be better and more regular.

★ ★ ★ ★ ★

The cocktail curse is stealing the health and life of thousands of our young men and women. You cannot acquire the habit of drinking alcoholic liquors and maintain the vitality and vigor that you should possess. You cannot be at your best depending on such stimulation.

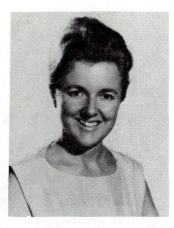

YOUR TONGUE
NEVER LIES

Your tongue is a "Magic Mirror". Your tongue can reveal how much toxic material is stored in the cells and vital organs of your body. The tongue is not only the mirror of the stomach, but the entire membrane system, as well.

In your body there is a hose-like tube that is 30 feet long, extending from the mouth to the anus. It has the body heat of 98.6 ... plus it has moisture. Through this tube passes all the food you eat. Now, different foods take different times to pass through the tube. The majority of people today eat a highly, refined, concentrated acid-forming diet. They eat large amounts of refined white flour, refined white sugar, and saturated fats. Most of these so-called civilized diets lack sufficient bulk, moisture, and lubrication to pass quickly through the 30-foot tube.

I believe that there is a common factor that precedes or is coexistent with the many ills that affect us. This common denominator is constipation. Definitions may differ, but, in my opinion, it is logical that if outgo does not equal intake, either in point of quantity or in frequency, then constipation occurs. Constipation can be the beginning of many serious physical problems.

In our culture, people are brainwashed to believe there is no harm in eating anything, and as often as it is desired. We are told to eat a huge breakfast to furnish plenty of energy for all morning, but then many people consume more food at a mid-morning coffee break. Then comes lunch, a midafternoon coffee break, the usual heavy evening meal, then T.V. snacks ... and a bedtime snack before retiring. On top of all this food, many people will gorge on ice cream, rich, thick malted milks, frozen treats on sticks, candy bars, and salted nuts. This means that food is ingested six or more times a day.

Now the average person believes that if they have one good
bowel movement a day, usually in the morning, that they are
free of constipation. One full bowel movement is not sufficient
to remove all of the food material these people are gorging
into their intestinal tracts, and as a consequence, this rotten,
putrifying, morbid waste, lies undischarged in the intestine,
where it undergoes enzymatic and bacteriological changes, that
often cause severe physical problems.

The human body is basically strong and can take a lot of abuse
from too much eating, and too much of the wrong kind of food.
It is most difficult to tell these people who eat incorrectly, and
have only one bowel movement a day, that they are constipated, and
thus inviting serious troubles later. But there is one warning
signal — an unhealthy tongue — that can tell these people they
are carrying a nasty cesspool within their bodies.

If these people fasted for two or three days on distilled water
exclusively, the tongue, the "Magic Mirror" would tell them
quite plainly that they are carrying a horrible mass of fer -
menting poison in the intestinal tube. A few days of fasting
will coat the tongue with a thick, white, rancid, toxic material
that has a terrible odor. This heavy coating of toxic material
can be scraped off and examined. In fast, you can scrape the
tongue clean, but, in a few hours, the heavy toxic coating will
return. It is an accurate indication of the amount of putrifying
toxic filth, mucus, and many other poisons accumulated in the
cells of your entire body, which is now being eliminated from
the inside surface of the stomach, intestines, and from all
parts and organs of the body.

The actual amount of toxic material that the average, so-called
healthy person carries around with him is almost unbelievable.
In my opinion, many physical problems are a special, local
constipation of the 30-foot intestinal tube, of the circulation,
cells, and the entire pipe system of the human body. I believe
that these poisons cause a constitutional clogging of the entire
human pipe system, especially the microscopically-small
capillaries.

By coating the tongue of the faster, Nature definitely shows
that his body contains a large amount of toxic poison. The
characteristics of tissue construction, especially of the powerful, vital, internal organs, such as the kidneys, liver, and all
glands, are like those of a sponge. Imagine a sponge filled
with a putrifying mass of thick paste. I have supervised hundreds of fasts, and only a person with my long experience
knows the great amount of toxic poison that lies in the body of
the average person who lives on the standard American diet.

Think of a simple illustration ... for instance, someone with a common cold ... Have you ever stopped to think how much mucus and phlegm passes out of the body through the nose and throat. This is also how the vital organs, such as the lungs, kidneys, and bladder are passing out poisons, during this cleansing crisis.

So, start right now to learn more about yourself by fasting and closely watching your tongue. The tongue is a spongy organ that accurately mirrors on its surface the health or ill-health of every other part of your body. The "Magic Mirror" can be a guiding star in your journey of Super-Health.

The more faithfully you follow a good fasting schedule ... the more accurately you follow a program of natural eating — the cleaner your tongue will become during a fast.

This is a definite signpost that you are on the Road to a New Life ... a life free of physical problems and misery ... a road that will lead to your greatest achievement — AGELESSNESS and a Painless, Ageless, Tireless Body! So, as you go on your 24-hour or 36-hour or 7- or 10-day fast, note how much cleaner your tongue will become with each fast. This will reveal to you the amazing Miracle of Fasting. Man does not die of old age ... it has been proven that there are no special diseases that are due simply to old age.

Most diseases kill the young as well as the aged. And many of these diseases are from a body loaded with toxic poisons. Keep the body clean by fasting and eating only wholesome, natural food. Your tongue and your urine can be your guideposts to internal purity. Watch both carefully as you fast.

★ ★ ★ ★ ★

LAW OF LIFE

Man's body was created according to the laws of physics and chemistry, which are the Creator's own laws. They never vary. His law is written upon every nerve, every muscle, every faculty, which has been entrusted to us.

These laws govern the cells, tissues, and organs of the body as they carry on their various functions. They operate largely through the complex network of nerves that run throughout the body. They act through the central nervous system, from which nerve impulses originate, and through the autonomic nervous system, that part of the network not under the direct control of the will.

-Henry W. Vollmer, M.D.

"I want to fast, because I believe it would do wonders for me, but how can I fast and yet escape the great feeling of hunger that the first three days of fasting produces?" That is the question that is put to me many, many times when I discuss the Miracle of Fasting at my Health lectures all over the world.

And I have only one answer "Just Grin and Bear ... "

"I tried a fast once, but I got so weak, and felt so miserable, I just had to start eating".

This is another statement I often hear.

Nowhere in this book have I stated that fasting is easy.

Eating has become such an important part of people's lives that if you take food away from them, and start them on a fast, they experience many mental and physical reactions. That is the very reason why fasting is not popular. Humans are creatures of habit. Most people automatically eat three or more meals every day, and not because they have earned their food by physical activity. They have been brainwashed to believe that everyone should have strict, regular hours of eating.

Recently I had the pleasure of staying at the fabulous new Rockefeller Hotel, The Mauna Kea, on the Island of Hawaii. It is an American plan hotel, which means the cost per day for your room includes meals ... breakfast was at 7:30 A.M., luncheon at 12:30 P.M., and dinner at 7 P.M. Whenever I passed the dining room at these hours, the guests were all eagerly waiting for the doors to open so they could get at the food.

★ ★ ★ ★ ★

The Doctor of the future will give no medicine but will interest his patients in the care of the human frame in diet and in the cause and prevention of disease.

- Thomas A. Edison

Were they hungry at exactly these hours? How could they be? Most of the guests did nothing but relax on the beach, or played cards or read. They had done absolutely nothing to earn these meals ... but they were there believing that they should eat their meals at regular times. It was the same on the ship when I returned home to California ... there was always a crowd of people waiting for the dining room doors to open.

DON'T LIVE TO EAT — EAT TO LIVE

Food! Food! Food! It can be a Blessing to mankind, but it also can be a curse. The human body can take a lot of abuse from overfeeding. But there comes a day when the body's digestive system refuses to overwork, and hundreds of terrible troubles start.

Digestive troubles plague civilized man. Constipation heads the list of his miseries. Tons upon tons of pills, powders, and liquids are sold to try and flush out the waste packed in the human intestines. Civilized man packs food into himself faster than the functions of digestion and elimination can handle. This is very much like trying to speed your car with the brakes on.

There is merit to the contention that constipation is the foundation for many other ailments.

The reason behind this contention is sound. If constipation means retention of intestinal waste, here is a very simple test you can make. Prepare your next meal, made up of everything you would ordinarily eat, but do not eat a mouthful of it. Instead, put it in a pot; place the container with the food in a temperature of around 100 degrees, the same as that inside the body. See that there is a liberal quantity of moisture. Now watch what takes place over the next eight hours.

The very first things you will notice are the bad odors and rancidity. Then the food will ferment and bubble with gas. This gas pressure can cause many miseries in the body. If the gas presses upward against the diaphragm; you may have stimulated a heart attack. As it presses against the back muscles, it causes a terrible aching back. When in the body, this fermenting mass of putrefaction is constantly throwing off toxins which can cause pounding headaches, and mysterious aches and pains all over the body.

Elementary bacteriology tells us that, to produce germs in quantity, keep food fermenting in the colon, and the bacteria will obligingly multiply. So, right in our bodies, we breed all kinds of "bugs" that can spread a lot of trouble.

If you are prone to any of the bacteriological ailments such as frequent colds, chronic sinusitis, and other ailments, a constipated condition creates a favorable environment for the presence and growth of unfriendly "bugs" involved in such ailments.

The toxic poison generated by too much food, and too much of the wrong kind of food, can damage one of the most important organs in the body, the liver. Few people realize how important the liver is to life. The liver is truly a great chemical laboratory, with many functions. It not only gives forth bile, but it is the body's greatest garbage disposal. The liver and intestines are partners in the whole digestive process. If one is sick, the other tries to come to its aid until it, too, breaks down. When the liver and the digestive systems break down, you are in serious trouble. This is why you often find, along with constipation, a swollen sensitive liver, a pasty complexion, and many times, jaundice and general debility.

So, it is plain that when you stop eating to give the Vital Force of the body a chance to clean house, you are bound to miss your food, so the first few days of the fast could be uncomfortable.

When you fast, the Vital Force loosens the waste in the body and sends it into the circulation to be discarded. As long as this goes on, you feel miserable. But, once the waste is discarded through the kidneys, you begin to feel much better. As you fast, conditions change from day to day. When the body is eliminating heavy amounts of toxic poisons through the kidneys and other organs of elimination, you feel wretched. But it should also be clear why you may feel better on the seventh day of a ten day fast than you did on the third day. These toxic poisons that gave you trouble have been flushed out of the body. Many fasters, under my supervision, felt far better and stronger on the tenth day of the fast than they did on the first day.

This always happens to me when I take a 7- or 10-day fast. I always feel stronger at the end of my fast than I did at the beginning. The cleaner you are inside, the more Vital Power you have. So, at the beginning of the fast, just grin and bear the discomforts that may occur as you purify the body. You know that, as you cleanse, you are going to feel stronger. Whatever discomforts you may experience during a fast are well worth the great rewards you are going to receive. Again I say, to be a good faster "Just Grin and Bear".

★ ★ ★ ★ ★

"Accuse not nature, she hath done her
part; do thou but thine."

- Milton, Paradise Lost

15

DEFEATING MUCUS BY RATIONAL FASTING

In my opinion most of man's problems stem from a clogging of the entire pipe system of the human body. Most of this clogging is in the form of a thick mucus.

At this minute, how free are you of mucus? Do you have a post-nasal drip, that is, is there a slow dripping of mucus from your sinus cavities dripping into the back of your mouth and throat? What about your nose? How much mucus are you carrying in the nose cavity? How many times a day do you use your hankerchief or paper tissue? How many times a day do you clear your throat? How many times a day do you raise mucus and phlegm?

Every person living on the average food of civilization has more or less a mucus-clogging pipe system. Such toxic mucus results from undigested and uneliminated, unnatural food substances, accumulated almost since birth. This mucus not only clogs the nose, throat, and lungs, but mucus can be found all along the 30 feet of the gastrointestinal tract that starts at the mouth and extends to the anus. Some humans suffer great distress from heavy mucus clogging in the sinus cavities. It is found in the ears, not only in liquid form, but cemented into a hardened wax. The greatest accumulation of mucus is found in the lungs.

Pneumonia is one of the most deadly of our diseases, and pneumonia invades our bodies when the lungs become so clogged with mucus that no oxygen, in the right amounts, can get into the lungs to purify the 5 to 8 quarts of blood which flow to the lungs for purification. Our bodies are equipped with an elastic pipe system.

The civilized diet that we eat is never entirely digested and accumulated waste never entirely eliminated. This entire pipe system is slowly but surely clogging, especially at the place of the symptom and the digestive tract. This is the foundation of many physical problems. The body is overloaded with mucus which the avenues of elimination cannot get rid of. It starts in the body and concentrates into a decayed mass.

★ ★ ★ ★ ★

Eat to live, and not live to eat

Many dishes, many diseases. – Ben Franklin

OUR CIVILIZED DIET FORMS MUCUS

The diet of civilization is a mucus-forming diet. Most civilized diets are made up of fried foods, and all fried foods are mucus-forming. Dairy products are highly mucus-forming. No animal in the world except man drinks milk after it is weaned. Civilized diet includes butter, butter substitutes, margarines, hydrogenated or hardened oils and fats which the body cannot metabolize. About 90 percent of all commercial shortenings are made from hydrogenated and hardened fats, known as the saturated fats. Our bodies have a normal temperature of 98.6. To digest and assimilate the hardened, saturated fats, our bodies would have to have a heat of 300 degrees. Our civilized diet contains a great deal of processed and synthetic cheese as well as natural cheeses which are heavily saturated with salt and I have discussed salt quite fully in this book.

Eggs are eaten extensively, yet eggs carry a large amount of saturated fats which are known as cholesterol. Our civilized diet calls for a lot of meat, most of it fried in heavy grease, either lard, or hydrogenated commercial oils. Meat also carries a heavy load of fat both visible and invisible. In our modern civilization, much of our cooking is done by the deep-fat method, such as French-fried potatoes, one of the most popular foods among civilized people. You can plainly see that the modern civilized diet is a mucus-forming diet.

MUCUS SHOWS UP IN THE URINE WHEN FASTING

The urine test is a truthful story of the amount of mucus that the average human carries within the blood stream. Take a 3-day fast, eat absolutely nothing, and drink only large amounts of distilled water from 2 to 3 quarts a day. Every morning of the fast, take a sample of the first urine you pass on awakening, put it in a bottle, place it on a shelf to cool and settle ... in a few days this urine will

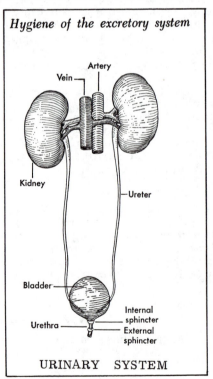

Hygiene of the excretory system

Artery

Vein

Kidney

Ureter

Bladder

Urethra

Internal sphincter

External sphincter

URINARY SYSTEM

show a heavy cloud of mucus. The longer you keep the urine, the more this cloud of urine will reveal itself. In my opinion, a 24-hour fast weekly will help you rid your body of large amounts of mucus. Some of this mucus has been circulating in your blood for years and years. In the wintertime, when people specialize in heavy, concentrated foods, such as pancakes, cereals, doughnuts, buns, bread, white rice, flour gravies, cakes and pies, the body will become so loaded with mucus that it will force the Vital Power to create a cleansing crisis. A fluid will be produced by the Vital Power to help burn up the heavy concentrations of mucus. The nose and throat will pour out large quantities of mucus. Few humans realize what a holocaust is going on in the body.

The body is a self-purifying instrument, and as long as the body has Vital Power to eliminate poisons such as mucus, it will work with all its energy to rid the body of this foreign fluid. But what do humans think about this crisis? They feel the fever. A fever is a natural phenomenon of nature. Dead people do not have fevers, it is only live people with lots of vitality who have the high fevers which act as Mother Nature's incinerator.

The poor ignorant man will tell you that because he got his feet wet, he is suffering this winter misery, or he will say that a draft blew on him, or he didn't get his sweater or coat on in time. These are weak and unscientific excuses. Winter miseries are Nature's effort to get rid of excess amounts of toxic mucus within the body chemistry. It is Nature's built-in purification and cleansing mechanism.

I have proven over and over that you can't catch anything. At the turn of the century, I was associated with Bernarr Macfadden, the father and founder of the Physical Culture Movement. He organized a group of people known as the Polar Bears, and every Saturday, Sunday, and holiday in the frigid winter weather, we would go to the beach at Coney Island, New York, and frolic and exercise on the beach. Then we would all plunge into the icy water of the Atlantic Ocean. Did I ever see one of the winter bathers even have the sniffles? Never! People would come to Coney Island bundled up in heavy overcoats, mufflers, sweaters and flannel underwear and stand on the boardwalk, staring at us, swimming and splashing around in the icy water. They were the people who had the sniffles, not the Polar Bears who believed in eating a mucusless diet, exercising heavily outdoors, and swimming in the icy waters of the Atlantic. Today I belong to two fine organizations who swim the year around at Coney Island, New York — the Polar Bears and the Icebergs. These two clubs are made up of men and women who are cold-water swimmers. I also belong to the Winter Bathers Club (The Boston Brownies) in Boston at the "L" Street Bath House.

Here is another group of men who prove that you can swim and expose yourself to the most frigid weather and still never have a sniffle, a chill, a fever, or other reactions from exposure to cold weather.

I live in California and the Pacific Ocean drops down to around 50 degrees in January, February, and March, and if I am not on a lecture tour in some other part of the world, you can count on me taking my daily cold water swims at the beach in Santa Monica where I have a home.

There are many of my friends, who live on a natural diet free from mucus-forming foods, who join me in my cold-water, winter bathing. I feel that fasting has done a great deal to eliminate the mucus from my body. Of course I try to live on a mucusless diet and I feel my weekly 24-hour fast helps me keep the mucus flowing outward that I may accumulate in my body.

Make the test yourself, eliminate all of the mucus-forming foods for several months ... fast one day a week and if possible take a seven-day fast. Watch your urine closely, see for yourself the amount of mucus you have concentrated in your blood stream. After a fast, make one-half of your diet raw vegetables, raw fruits, and cooked non-starchy vegetables. This is a mucusless diet. Nuts and seeds are not mucus-forming, so to the diet of raw fruits and vegetables, and cooked fruit and vegetables, you may add sunflower seeds, sesame seeds, unsalted nut butters, and any kind of nuts. If you eat meat and fish, limit it to not over three times a week, and you should not eat over three eggs weekly. Go lightly on whole-grains, cereals, and breads. I do not have to tell you what fasting and a mucusless diet will do for you, simply try it yourself. You be the judge ... study your urine, see how very seldom you have to use a hankerchief or tissue. A seven-day fast is a great mucus-eliminator. I make it a practice to fast a week to ten days in late October or November so that as the winter comes on, I have relieved my body of any mucus that may have accumulated. I try to live on a mucusless diet, but while traveling all over the world, lecturing, I find that at times I cannot get the amount of fruits and vegetables that I normally use, so I put my faith in fasting for internal purification.

BREAKING THE TOBACCO, ALCOHOL, TEA, AND COFFEE HABIT THROUGH FASTING

Most humans in civilization are addicted to some kind of drug poisoning. Tobacco, alcohol, tea, and coffee are drug habits. Every one of these substances have dangerous toxic poisons. The spotlight of science has been focused on the use of tobacco for a long time to the point, that on every package of cigarettes the following warning will be given "tobacco may be a health hazard". Great Scientists around the world have investigated the effect of tobacco on human flesh. Again let me reiterate ... "FLESH IS DUMB" — "FLESH WILL ACCEPT ANYTHING".

It will accept the carbon monoxide and nicotine of tobacco, and will accept alcohol. It will accept the caffeine tars found in coffee and tea. The human body has no mechanism to handle these vicious drugs and poisons ... but man seems to have a desire to destroy himself, in spite of all the research pointing out the dangers!

Now, if a person wishes to release himself from the bondage of these irritating stimulants which we call depressants, these drugs act first to stimulate, and then to depress the central nervous system.

The fast is a salvation for the man or woman who wishes to break the shackles of these poisonous habits. In many years of supervising fasts, I have seen these wretched habits defeated through fasting.

I remember several years ago a woman came to me who was a chain-smoker. She smoked at least 4 packages of cigarettes a day ... she consumed at least a fifth of whisky daily, and was a heavy user of coffee and tea. She told me her central nervous system was a shambling wreck. If she picked up a pencil to write, she trembled. She couldn't sleep, her appetite was gone ... her eyes were blurred, her skin-tone was pasty and flabby.

She was so miserable, she had even turned to thoughts of self-destruction. Her physician suggested that she see me, that through physical therapy, I might give her some relief. She was willing to try anything. She had reached the end of her rope.

The first thing I did was to start her on a fast, I did not take her poison away from her, so she continued to smoke, and drank a small amount of alcohol and coffee, but on the morning of the third day of the fast, her body rebelled and these poisons that she had so frequently used began to nauseate her. Every time she would light a cigarette, every time she would take a small amount of alcohol or coffee, she had heavy attacks of vomiting. I supervised the fast for ten days. This was the first seven days for many years that she had not polluted and degenerated her body with these deadly poisons. I broke her fast on the tenth day and the urine that she passed on the tenth morning was a thick mass of ugly material. You know what this material was — the residue of her poisons. I put her on a mucus-less diet for ten days and then fasted her again for ten days. Every day of the 2nd ten-day fast, large amounts of toxic poisons showed in the urine. She stayed under my supervision for ten months.

I had her photographed at the beginning of the program and at the end of ten months, and you would hardly know it was the same woman. Her skin and muscle-tone were perfect, her hands were firm and steady. Instead of a miserable, depressed human, she was now a happy and carefree person! She has never had the desire for tobacco, alcohol, tea, or coffee, and today she is one of the most outstanding writers in the demanding Hollywood T.V. and movie world. Her income has doubled and tripled, her personal magnetism increased to such an extent that she attracted a handsome and wholesome man for a husband.

I could give you many other instances of people who had hit the bottom in their addictions of tobacco, alcohol, tea, and coffee, but turned to fasting as a last resort and fasting did the trick. Any person who is addicted to tobacco, alcohol, tea, and coffee will find an answer to their problem simply by fasting. When the body becomes clean, it will no longer allow poisons to enter. A pure, clean, and wholesome body will always reject poisons of any kind. Fasting is the greatest method known for purifying the body so that it sets up an active resistance to any poisons that try to enter the body.

★ ★ ★ ★ ★

"Living under conditions of modern life, it is important to bear in mind that the preparation and refinement of food products either entirely eliminates or in part destroys the vital elements in the original material."

United States Government
Dept. of Agriculture

★

If your food is devitalized, the important elements of nourishment have been removed, or if its value has been diminished by the cooking process,--you can then starve to death on a full stomach.

16

FASTING HELPS POUNDS MELT AWAY

It is estimated on good authority that 65 to 70 percent of men, women, and children in our country are overweight. An overweight person is in serious condition, as we are told by the greatest medical authorities and insurance companies. Overweight can be a great hazard to health and long-life. These authorities tell us that the overweight person is much more susceptible to many chronic and even fatal diseases. An overweight person cannot begin to feel the thrill of well-being. First, they are constantly tired because they are carrying far too many pounds. Let us say that a person is 25 pounds overweight. Now, let's ask a normal person to carry a 25-pound weight around all day. In a very short time every move would become painful and most fatiguing, so you can plainly see that an overweight person is really carrying an enormous burden that is equal to the number of pounds that they are overweight.

The fat person has no ambition to indulge in physical activities — most of them would rather find the closest chair and sit in it until they are forced to do some important duty. In fact, they have to almost beat themselves to do the things they have to do. The overweight person has a difficult time breathing because the excess flesh makes it very difficult for the organs of respiration to do their job properly, so we find them panting and puffing at the least exertion.

OVERWEIGHT IS A TREMENDOUS BURDEN

For every cubic inch of fat on the overweight person, the body must have 700 miles (unbelievable, but true) of fine tubes to nourish and sustain this excess fat. You can plainly see why the overweight person is putting a tremendous burden on the breathing apparatus, and the normal function of the heart. The pulse and blood pressure are forced to rise to dangerous heights, which could in itself bring on serious damage to the body — even death.

Insurance figures show accurately that overweight people are short-lived people and, as stated, they are susceptible to many chronic diseases because of this abnormal overweight condition. Any way you look at it, overweight is dangerous.

Today, overweight is steadily on the increase. First, in our country we have an abundance of food, and the average American loads large quantities of food into his stomach for the shear joy of eating. Eating is one of the indoor and outdoor sports of America. Family gatherings call for a table loaded with many varieties of food. When people entertain their relatives and friends there is always a tendency for over-eating due to far too many items of foods in the meal that has been planned.

Our coffee-breaks encourage people to snack between meals ... radio and television invite people to snack as they gaze into the idiot box. People are constantly swilling thick malted milks, ice cream, hot dogs, hamburgers, French-fried potatoes, pizza pie and many other varieties of food between meals. Then, too, banquets, benefit dinners, and buffet dinners, with far too much food and drink, encourage overeating.

We live in a mechanical age. We load heavy amounts of food into our bodies and never burn it up with exercise and physical activities. The automobile has replaced walking. We are a nation of sitters. Our children sit for hours in school. People spend hours attending movies, concerts, athletic events, musicals ... all this sedentary life increases the overweight of the average person.

THE AMERICAN CRASH DIETS

Overweight people are constantly going on crash diets of some kind. There is the high-protein diet, the low-carbohydrate diet, the Air Force diet, the pineapple and lamb chop diet, the egg and tomato diet. Magazine after magazine, newspaper after newspaper, are always blurting some new sensational crash diet to take weight off the obese person. There are liquid diets which advise people to drink 800 calories a day ... there are the cottage cheese diets, the low-fat milk diet ... there are so many reducing diets, that it is frustrating and confusing to know which one to follow. In my opinion, the fast is the only natural and scientific way for reasonable reduction in weight. Let me give you some of my reasons why I believe fasting is the perfect way to reduce.

After the first 2 or 3 days of fasting you are no longer hungry ... from the third day on, there is no craving for food. When people go on special diets that are generally low-calorie diets, they are miserable and hungry most of the time. They become obsessed, longing for heavy meals, but after you fast for 2 or 3 days, all hunger fades away, the stomach shrinks, and it actually becomes a very pleasant experience. You start to breathe easier; you have greater freedom of movement; and you completely lose that washed-out, dragged-out feeling.

★ ★ ★ ★ ★

"Tell me what you eat and I will tell you want you are."

FASTING REWARDS YOU WITH INCREASED ENERGY

I have seen many overweight people lose 7 to 12 pounds of weight
the first 7 to 10 days of fasting. With the loss of this excess
weight, there is a certain inner-feeling of well-being and increased energy...a lightness comes over the body, a feeling of
buoyancy. Of course, every human is different. Some people
only lose 1 or 2 pounds a day on a fast, while as I have stated,
some will lose as many as 5 pounds. The nice thing about fasting to reduce is that the pounds diminish where the fat is deposited. If the weight has concentrated on the abdomen and hips,
that is where the fat will shrink. Many times, people who go on
a low-calorie diet, feeling miserable while they are dieting, will
become haggard and old looking...their eyes will lose their
sparkle, but when you fast, it is just the reverse. The fat spots
dissolve first, and as the body is relieved of this tremendous
burden, the heart, pulse, and blood pressure will regulate itself.

So, if you have a weight problem, use the Fasting Program as
outlined in this book. You can start with a 24-hour fast weekly.
I often supervise weight-reducing programs, where I direct persons to fast from 1 to 3, 24-hour periods a week...in other words,
they will eat one day and fast the next day. If the person does
not overload himself on the days he eats, the 36-hour fast several times a week will retain his loss of weight. Fasting for
weight reduction gets substantial results of weight loss. Your
body slims and trims itself back to youthful lines again.

I have had years of experience in fasting many of our greatest
film and television stars in Hollywood, California. The movie
camera always makes a person look 10 pounds heavier than he
really is, so you can see that a star must always have slim,
trim lines. The waistline is your lifeline and also your dateline!

I recall a few years ago, a well-known feminine movie star who
became a compulsory eater because she was having marital and
financial troubles. She sought solace in eating, particularly
rich foods, such as ice cream, heavily-sugared pastries, and
candies. In time she lost her movie contract because she was
just an ugly, fat woman. She was a good actress, but the public
makes severe demands on their public favorites. This woman
became depressed and had to seek the services of a psychiatrist.
The psychiatrist sent this actress to me for physiotherapy. When
she came to me, I explained that it had taken time for her to add
this weight on her body, and that it would take time to slim, trim,
and normalize the fat. She was determined to lose weight, so I
had a student who was most cooperative.

I will call this lady, "Betty", although that is not her name.
Betty was about 50 pounds overweight. First, I put her on a

good diet program, with fruit for breakfast, a raw salad with two (5-percent) cooked vegetables for lunch, such as string beans, cooked celery, spinach, stewed tomatoes or squash. I took all bread, cereals, rice and potatoes out of her diet. In the evening she had lettuce and tomatoes, a piece of broiled fish or a hard boiled egg or one lamb chop. Naturally, all desserts were eliminated from the diet. I started her on two, 24-hour fasts a week for the first two weeks, the third week I gave her a 3-day fast, the fifth week I gave her a full 7-day fast. After one week of eating, as stated above, I put her on a 15-day fast, then I fed her for two weeks and put her on a 21-day fast. This eating and fasting program did the trick. Her girlish figure returned, her eyes became bright and clear and her skin and muscle tone had the appearance of youthfulness. Producers and directors were amazed at her transformation.

Through sensible fasting and intelligent dieting, she now has attained her normal weight of 110 pounds for a height of 5'2''. She continues with her diet and takes one 36-hour fast every week and a 7-day fast four times a year, spaced at 3-month intervals. If there is such a thing as retaining youthful beauty and a stream-lined body, fasting is the magic formula.

BUT, REMEMBER, FASTING IS A CHALLENGE

Our eating habits are so ingrained in our consciousness that fasting to many humans is starvation. It is not starvation...fasting is one of the oldest remedies of man, but again I say, the mind must control the flesh. "FLESH IS DUMB".

It takes intelligence and logic and reasoning to know when to turn down food. If you are a determined person, if you believe in the law of compensation, you will make fasting an important part of your life. Don't let overweight make you a sick, old, ugly person. Revolt against fat, be the master of your body. Say to yourself, I am no longer going to be burdened with ugly, sick, flabby flesh. Work out a program for yourself, and don't try to get the fat off in one week. It took a long time to get there and it will take a reasonable length of time to melt away. You will be so proud of yourself when you slim and trim yourself down to your normal weight and normal measurements.

Every man and woman is born with pride and vanity, we all want to look our best, we all want to feel our best, so let's do something about it! Fasting and sensible, sane dieting is your answer! Be sure you have a bathroom scale and get yourself a tape measure. Weigh yourself and measure abdomen, hips, thighs, and arms. With determination and the knowledge you have learned of fasting in this book, steel yourself to a serious program of weight-reduction.

To prove the value of fasting, go to your doctor and get a physical examination before you start your fasting program. After the program has been completed and you have reached your goal, you will be amazed at the marvelous benefits that you have received from your Fasting Program. I know that the doctor will even congratulate you on your achievements.

There is no easy way to take off fat, and I am not going to tell you fasting is easy. It is going to take Positive Thinking, and Positive Action, to attain Positive Results! Start today to lose those dangerous excess pounds!

IMPORTANT EXERCISES FOR KEEPING THE EXTERNAL
AND THE INTERNAL MUSCLES OF THE ABDOMEN -
FIRM AND HEALTHY.

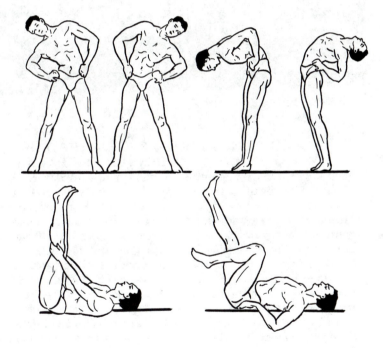

Weakness of the muscles of the arms and legs and
other parts of the body indicates a similar condition
of the muscles of the heart, stomach and other organs.

WHEN YOU ARE HEALTHY — YOU ARE HAPPY!

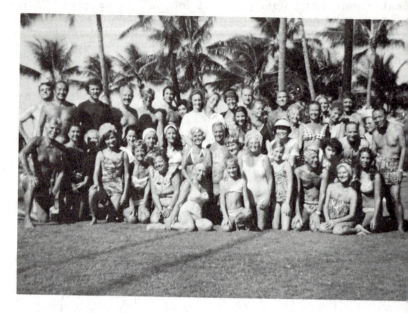

JOIN THE FUN AT THE "LONGER LIFE, HEALTH AND HAPPINESS CLUB" WHEN YOU VISIT HAWAII

Paul and Patricia Bragg and some of their prize members of the "Longer Life, Health and Happiness Club" at their exercise compound at Fort DeRussy, right at Waikiki Beach, Honolulu, Hawaii. Membership is free and open to everyone who wishes to attend any morning Monday through Saturday from 8:30 a.m. to 10:30 a.m. for deep breathing, exercising, meditation, group singing and mini health lectures on how to live a long, healthy life! The group averages 75 to 100 per day. When they are away lecturing they have their leaders carry on until their return. Thousands have visited the club from around the world and then they carry the message of health and happiness to their friends and relatives back home. Paul and Patricia extend an invitation to you and your friends to join the club for health and happiness fellowship with them . . . when you visit Hawaii!

SCIENTIFIC FASTING *PROGRAM*

Skinny, emaciated, people fight frantically to gain and hold a few pounds. Gaining weight becomes an obsession with the underweight person, and they are most susceptible to all kinds of weight-gaining diets. Underweight people have come to me in a frustrated and emotional condition, begging me to help them to put a few pounds on their sparse frames. Most of them were cold constantly, and even on the warmest summer days they wore sweaters and heavy garments. They begged me to give them a diet that would help them gain weight, because they were ashamed of their skeleton-like bodies.

When I told them there was no such a thing as a weight-gaining diet, they were as shocked as if I had given them a death sentence. But, when I added most emphatically that there was a program to gain weight which included fasting, they would agree on the program, but not on the fasting. They would cry out, "Don't make me any thinner than I am! I am down to skin and bones now, but if you take my food away from me, I will look like a scarecrow". Then I had to explain that they were thin only because their bodies were off-balance nutritionally. I told them that food and nutrition are not synonymous, and that I could formulate a diet that was rich in fats, carbohydrates, and sugar ... I could add gallons of milk, cream, and more fattening foods, but that wouldn't help them to gain weight. The body would get thinner carrying this load.

People are not nourished in proportion to the amount of food they eat, but in proportion to how much they digest and assimilate. When the organs of digestion and assimilation are in poor working condition, eating too many fat foods to gain weight defeats its own purpose.

Underweight is due to impairment of the general health of the person. It is futile to stuff a lot of food into the body when assimilation and digestion are working at a low ebb. The secret of gaining weight is to make the detoxifying system more efficient by fasting. Then the underweight person rejuvenates the digestive and assimilative system of the body.

What the underweight person needs is exactly what the overweight person needs — a fast — which gives the body a physiological rest. In both the overweight and the underweight, the digestive system and assimilation system of the human body has been overworked. This is difficult to explain to underweight and emaciated persons. They are impatient and want to gain weight immediately on a diet, but, first, the underweight person must realize that the period of physiological rest provided by the fast results in better digestion and assimilation of foods. The body has extraordinary recuperative powers when it is not burdened with an excess amount of food. In over 50 years of fasting underweight people, I have had outstanding success with underweight and emaciated people who learned to have faith in fasting and a full program of natural living.

I have a sister whom I love very dearly and who was born a very tiny baby. I believe, if I am correct, she weighed about 3 pounds. All through her life, my sister Louise was called "skinny" and when she was a child, everyone would tell my mother that she should be stuffed with milk and cream, and that she must eat a lot of pork, potatoes, rice, custards and all the supposed weight-gaining foods, but the more my sister was stuffed with all of these so-called fattening foods, the thinner, the weaker, the paler, and the more lifeless she became. There were many times when my sister was so weak that she had to remain in bed, but even during these periods in bed, she was still stuffed on a so-called weight-gaining diet.

Later, after I had left home, and after regaining my health, I returned to Virginia, where my sister Louise lived. She was now an adult and unmarried. She was teaching high school and was a thin, emaciated, run-down, weak-looking person. Her color was ghastly and after a hard day in the class room, she would come home and throw herself across the bed in a state of exhaustion, so tired she would weep.

I wrote her that I had found a natural way for people to gain weight and, when school closed and summer vacation began, I would return to Virginia and supervise a program to help her gain weight. She had seen the great miracle that had happened to my body by living the natural life...and had perfect confidence in everything I told her. I explained to her that part of the program would be a series of fasts, which would give her body a physiological rest and let the digestive and the assimilative organs of her body have a chance to revivify and rejuvenate. This is a system of detoxication, and I told her that the fast would help increase the hydrochloric acid in her stomach so that she could absorb more protein foods. Not only would the digestion of protein be better, but all the digestive organs would improve and renew themselves through the fast. Her whole process of metabolism (the sum of the processes concerned in the building up of protoplasm and its destruction incidental to life; the chemical changes in living cells, by which the energy is provided for the vital processes and activities, and new material is assimilated to repair the waste) would improve her fasting program.

I have proved over the years that when metabolism is improved by fasting, there is a great density, a specific gravity in the new flesh that is built after fasting. The fast assists the body to assimilate proteins, fats, carbohydrates, starches, sugars, minerals, and vitamins and all essential nutrients necessary for the body to work efficiently.

I started Louise on a 7-day distilled water fast. She entered this fast believing that Nature was going to purify her body, purify her digestive and assimilative organs, and help her rebuild a new body. It is true that she lost weight in the 7 days of the fast, but after I broke the fast, what a hardy, healthy, appetite she developed. What wonders this week's rest of the digestive and assimilating organs did for her. She told me she had never enjoyed food as much as she now was enjoying her new diet, not of the so-called "good nourishing, fattening food", but a diet of 50 percent of fresh, raw vegetables and luscious, fresh fruits. Along with raw fruits and vegetables, I gave her cooked vegetables, sun-flower meal, sesame meal, wheat germ, nuts and nut-butters of all kinds. In 3 weeks after the first fast, I gave her another fast of 10 days and this 10-day fast started a new life for her, because her body was in such fine condition that it started to round out.

My skinny, emaciated, sister, became a beautiful woman... rounded and stream-lined, and every part of her body seemed to be rejuvenated. Her hair took on a sheen it never had before, there was a glow to her cheeks, and a sparkle in her eyes that only a young baby has. Our relatives, friends, and neighbors were flabbergasted at the transformation in Louise. The happiest part of the whole matter is that within a year, my sister was one of the most popular girls in Westmoreland County, Virginia and in another year she married a fine handsome man. Their lives read like a fairy-tale because they had children, lived happily ever after. My sister retained her charm and beauty for many, many years.

Along with fasting, I gave my sister a system of exercises. She started with short walks and then built up to long walks...I persuaded her to get an abundance of fresh air, take sun-baths and do at least 20 minutes of deep breathing daily...At all times, she maintained a tranquil and serene mind, because she worked with Nature and not against Nature.

What I did for my thin sister, I have done with hundreds of under-weight people. Fasting works wonders for both the overweight and the thin. The genuine needs for both types of people are exactly the same program of natural living combined with fasting.

Fasting is the magic key for helping anyone to restore themselves to a superior state of health. Fasting is the great detoxifier and in detoxifying the body we give it a chance to be normal in its functioning. Fasting is the great "Open Sesame" to good health and long life.

Each person is different, and some get results more quickly than others, but if you really concentrate on a program of natural living in which fasting is an important part, Nature will never fail you.

So, if you are thin and underweight and have tried all sorts of weight-building diets that failed, do not be discouraged until you try a program of fasting. Give Nature a chance to make you a person of normal weight.

★ ★ ★ ★ ★

Credo of the famous Buchinger Clinics in Germany and Spain:

> "We must restore fasting to the place it occupied in an ancient hierarchy of values "above medicine." We must rediscover it and restore it to honor because it is a necessity. A beneficial fast of several weeks, as practiced in the earliest days of the Church, was to give strength, life, and health to the body and soul of all Christians who had the courage to practice it."

> *Christian Century* magazine advised its readers to fast out of enlightened self-interest and the objective to improve health, and make the body more vibrant and beautiful. "Fast because it is good for you," the magazine urged; it can be an "exercise to get the body in shape to be alive to itself. This process frees the self to be more sensitive to the Creation and to ourselves."

The Endless Quest

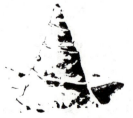

Freedom and progress rest in man's continual search for truth. Truth is the summit of being.   —Emerson

18

FIGHT THE SNIFFLES AND WINTER MISERIES WITH FASTING

No matter how well and wholesomely we try to live...once in awhile the sniffles will catch up with us. If this happens, please do not be discouraged with your Health program of living.

When your nose drips hot, burning, watery mucus and your head feels thick, you sneeze, fever burns through your body and you feel terrible, don't blame it on the weather...don't blame it on a cold draft of air...don't blame it on the fact that you got your feet wet...or that you got chilled. And above all things, don't say, "I CAUGHT IT". The proper name for this is an "acute healing crisis". The reason we go through this is that we live in a complex civilization, and we have lost so much of our natural instinct to keep internally pure.

So, for some physiological reason that is absolutely unexplainable, the Vital Force within our bodies loosens up waste and toxic matter and proceeds to get rid of it by the "acute healing crisis". If you will cooperate with your Vital Force, this rough spot in your life will pass away quickly. So, don't blame it on a vicious little bug, or a virus, or a draft. Just understand that the Vital Force is working on internal cleansing for YOU.

If you interfere with Nature, you will complicate the whole procedure of Nature's miraculous cleansing job. Now that you know what this acute healing crisis is, you should do nothing to stop the cleansing process - except to "FAST"...yes, that's the simple answer. F A S T!

Don't fight this healing crisis because Nature knows exactly what she is doing for you. What should you do? Get off your feet at once. There is absolutely nothing as important as your health and life. Drop everything you are doing and get into a warm bed ...stop all eating...that also means no fruit or fruit juices. At intervals, drink large amounts of hot distilled water with just a trace of honey and lemon juice. Nothing else. See that you have a good circulation of pure air in your bedroom. Don't read, don't listen to the radio, and don't watch T. V....just sleep and rest...nothing else. And, above all, don't waste your precious energy talking to relatives and friends. Go into complete seclusion.

How long should you fast for a winter healing crisis or, for that matter, a summer healing crisis? They can happen at any time of the year, but generally in cold weather. In most instances, three days will put you on your feet again. But sometimes it may take a week or ten days to do a successful job. Don't quibble about it...you will find that you are in better health after the healing crisis. If you will work with this Vital Force, you will flush out a tremendous amount of internal poisons. Just don't panic...Nature is so very wise and she knows what is best for you.

If you have faith and confidence in Nature, you will work with her. I reared five children and when the sniffles hit them...off to bed they went - fasting and resting. In a few days, they would snap out of the healing crisis and be their same robust selves again. My twelve grandchildren followed this program...and now my eight great-grandchildren are following it also! To most people this program seems too simple... THEY FEEL THAT THEY MUST DO SOMETHING or TAKE SOMETHING. They are filled with fear.

There is absolutely nothing to fear as long as Mother Nature is working to keep you alive and healthy. Mother Nature knows best and she will see you through any crisis, because she is God's physician.

Each person should regard his health as the most precious temporal blessing that he can possess and should attempt to understand his body which is so "fearfully and wonderfully made". He should maintain it in Supreme health, because that is far more important than a knowledge of all the arts.

Every man is not only the "Master Builder" of his character, but he is also the custodian of his health and physical well-being.

Not only has the Creator endowed man with a "God-Like" body; but he has given him a wonderful mind and the reasoning power capable of comprehending and putting to use natural resources for health and healing which have been so generously placed at his disposal. Fasting is just another way to Help Yourself to Greater Health. Nature gives us simple healing remedies. We must be willing to cooperate with Nature and conform our lives to Her immutable laws; and, through the "Natural Way of Living" we can recapture the precious boon of physical, mental, and spiritual regeneration. There are no short cuts to health. Nature expects us to do our part. When you fast you are working with Nature. God and Nature cannot and will not perform a miracle until we are willing to bring our lives and our habits into conformity with Nature's Laws.

★ ★ ★ ★ ★

"Everything in excess is opposed by Nature."

- Hippocrates

LET NATURE DO IT

It is my honest and sincere belief that no man should ever promise to cure anyone of any physical misery. To promise anyone a cure means that that man is playing God and Nature, and no man has the right to assume that grave responsibility.

By fasting, by eating only natural foods, and with other natural assistance, anyone can attain a more healthful life. Healing is an internal, biological function that only the body can perform, and by fasting you are helping your body do its work efficiently. Nature is continually working to keep you alive and well. So when Nature starts a healing crisis, she knows what she is doing. Go along with Nature, because she will never fail you.

Fasting is the greatest assistance you can give Nature, because you are letting her use all of your Vital Force to fight the toxic poisons and flush them out of your body.

★ ★ ★ ★ ★

WE THANK THEE

For flowers that bloom about our feet;
  For song of bird and hum of bee;
For all things fair we hear or see,
  Father in heaven we thank Thee!
For blue of stream and blue of sky;
  For pleasant shade of branches high;
For fragrant air and cooling breeze;
  For beauty of the blooming trees,
Father in heaven, we thank Thee!
  For mother-love and father-care,
For brothers strong and sisters fair;
  For love at home and here each day;
For guidance lest we go astray,
  Father in heaven, we thank Thee!
For this new morning with its light;
  For rest and shelter of the night;
For health and food, for love and friends;
  For every thing His goodness sends,
Father in heaven, we thank Thee!
                — Ralph Waldo Emerson

TOTAL HEALTH FOR THE TOTAL PERSON

In a broad sense, "Total Health for the Total Person" is a combination of physical, mental, emotional, social, and spiritual components. The ability of the individual to function effectively in his environment depends on how smoothly these components function as a whole. Of all the qualities that comprise an integrated personality, a well-developed, totally fit body is one of the most desirable.

A person may be said to be totally physically fit if they function as a total personality with efficiency and without pain or discomfort of any kind. That is to have a Painless, Tireless, Ageless body, possessing sufficient muscular strength and endurance to maintain an effective posture, successfully carries on the duties imposed by the environment, meets emergencies satisfactorily and has enough energy for recreation and social obligations after the "work day" has ended, meets the requirements for his environment through efficient functioning of his sense organs, possesses the resilience to recover rapidly from fatigue, tension, stress and strain without the aid of stimulants, and enjoys natural sleep at night and feels fit and alert in the morning for the job ahead.

Keeping the body totally fit and functional is no job for the uninformed or the careless person. It requires an understanding of the body, sound health and eating practices, and disciplined living. The results of such a regimen can be measured in happiness, radiant health, agelessness, peace of mind, in the joy of living and high achievement.

Paul C. Bragg and Patricia Bragg

"I have found a perfect health, a new state of existence, a feeling of purity and happiness, something unknown to humans . . ."
—Novelist Upton Sinclair,
who fasted frequently.

19

OUTWITTING PREMATURE AGEING WITH FASTING

YOUR MIRROR NEVER LIES

Go to your mirror now and take a good look at yourself. Are you happy with what you see? Do you look old and haggard? Does your face sag? Do you have poor skin tone? Do you have poor muscle tone? Is your face lined and wrinkled? Is your neck crepey? Are your eyes dull? Do you have a pale and sallow complexion?

After you have made a careful examination of your face, how would you describe it? Youthful? Aging? No one can answer these questions more honestly than you. You are the only person that can do something about it right now!

Let us go farther than mere looks. How do you really feel today? Are you bursting with energy and vitality? Or do you have bothersome aches and pains? What about the movable joints of your body? Are you stiff and sore? Does your lower back plague you with pain? How did you sleep last night? Did you get up fresh and feeling alive? Or did you go to bed tired, yet unable to sleep? Did you have a restless night? Did you face the new day feeling like a dishrag as if all your energy had drained away? How is your appetite? Do you relish every mouthful of food you eat? Were you plagued with gas pains after any of your meals today?

And what about your elimination? Was it perfect? Or are your bowels clogged?

And, above all things, were you happy today? And yesterday? Or were you depressed and blue?

Do you feel that you are aging rapidly and that life is slipping by?

Can you honestly and sincerely say "I am getting younger as I live longer"? Or will you have to admit that the longer you live, the older you feel? I am absolutely certain that you want to look young, that you yearn to feel young, I know that you hate the expression "I am getting old before my time".

Let me tell you honestly what fasting can do for you. This Nature miracle can help reverse the premature aging process for you. From this minute on, you could take a new lease on life. It has been proven by some of the world's greatest scientists that fasting is the magic key that opens the door to agelessness.

Scientists have been experimenting for years on worms, white rats, and guinea pigs, and they have discovered some remarkable scientific facts. They fasted these laboratory animals, and in between fasts they gave them scientifically-balanced, natural diets. A miracle occurred that sounds like a fairy tale - they got younger! It may seem too good to be true, but these scientists are single-minded and want only facts, and the facts revealed the truth. All these findings have been published and you need only go to a good library to read of these miraculous, vital discoveries.

Fasting not only holds back the clock, but it produces miraculous changes in the human body. In many years of fasting supervision, I have seen things happen to prematurely-old people that were almost unbelievable.

I remember a student of mine named Martin Cornica. Mr. Cornica had spent many years in the moving picture industry. He was about forty when he realized that he was aging prematurely, in fact, he regarded himself as a middle-aged man. And why shouldn't he? The average life expectancy of an American male today is 68 years of age, so he decided that at 40 he had lived over half his life, so he slowed his pace to that of a typical middle-aged man. There was once a time when Mr. Cornica was a champion tennis player, but he had long ago discarded his tennis racket, because obviously the game was only for the very young. Someone at 20th Century told Mr. Cornica about my Health Lectures. Out of sheer curiosity Mr. Cornica attended one of my Health Lectures.

That Lecture was a turning point in Mr. Cornica's life. He learned the same facts that I have given to thousands of people all over the world. When you know the science of taking care of the body, you have the secret of life. Mr. Cornica wanted to look and feel youthful. He was eager to try Nature's plan of living as I taught it.

He went on a 24-hour fast the day after he heard my health lecture. He began to eat a natural, wholesome perfectly balanced diet. With fasting and Natural living he dropped years from his age. Even though he was forty years old and regarded as long past the age to play strenuous tennis, Mr. Cornica felt stronger than when he was 20...his energy and vitality was temendous... so he joined the Los Angeles Tennis Club and started to play again. He still continued to fast and live on a Natural food diet, following the laws of hygiene, and every day, he improved in every way. His endurance was so strong that soon he was playing the champion tennis players of the world. For the next 30 years of his life, he played in one great tournament after another, and won championship after championship. Tennis is thought of as a game for only the young and vigorous, but here was a man supposedly long past the tennis age...playing with young champions, and winning.

TODAY MR. CORNICA IS THE WORLD'S CHAMPION TENNIS PLAYER OF THE WORLD FOR ALL MEN OVER 70. People in the tennis world are completely amazed when they see this man in his 70's playing a smashing, championship tennis game. They call him a "Freak".

The average person believes that by the time a man is seventy, he is either half-dead or absolutely dead, or a fumbling, doddering, broken old man. Mr. Cornica is the living proof of this fallacy. It is not the number of years you live on this earth... it is how you have lived! I am very proud of Mr. Cornica because he has absolutely proved that anyone can attain AGELESSNESS by following God's Natural Laws of Living.

Regardless of your age, Mother Nature will give you the opportunity to make a complete comeback...yes, you can step out of that old, wornout body of yours as you rebuild a body that will be AGELESS!

After a year of periodic fasting combined with a Natural Living Program, you can look at your mirror squarely, and be mighty happy with the tremendous improvement you have made in a mere years time. If you continue to live the life as programmed in this book, the transformation will make your friends and relatives sit up and marvel at your wonderful rejuvenation. You will not only see the difference in yourself...you will feel the difference. But, you can only make this transformation if you are willing to take over absolute mastery of your body.

Start as Mr. Cornica did with a 24-hour fast...read the chapter on correct eating in this book...call on the 8 doctors of Nature for aid in your program of rebirth. They are always ready and willing to help those who help themselves.

There is just one sad note that I must mention. As you get younger and more vital, you will see those you love the most begin to decay and pass out of life long before their time, because they refused to learn the "greatest law of life," which is "The Survival of the Fittest." The same thing has happened in my personal life. I have had to watch the people I loved the most, sicken, suffer, and die long before their time simply because they would not live a Natural Life.

★ ★ ★ ★ ★

"A strong body makes the mind strong."

- Writings of Thomas Jefferson

THE OPPORTUNITY OF YOUR LIFETIME

Revolt! Refuse to grow old! Refuse to lose precious years of your life! Mother Nature is waiting for you to make your decision this minute!

Good! You have decided to take the Health and Happiness road to Higher Health. There will be a few rough spots as you begin, but soon you will be hiking along the Highway of Health and Long-Lasting Youthfulness!

You cannot miss... you are working with God and Nature and these are forces that will never, ever fail you. Begin your 24-hour fast today. You will laugh at birthdays. They will mean nothing to you. You are living in the consciousness of Agelessness.

★ ★ ★ ★ ★

It is strange that any who believe in the biblical revelation should ever have thought that a practice so scriptural as fasting, taught and exemplified by Christ Himself, could ever be harmful to the body, provided it is carried out in accordance with Scripture. The fact is that the very reverse is the case. Fasting makes possible a process of physical therapy. It fully releases the body to operate its own natural system of cleansing and healing.

The loss of appetite, so often the first warning of the approach of acute illness, is thus not only a danger signal, but a signpost, pointing the way to recovery. It says in effect, 'Stop eating and give your body a chance to recover'.

The curative power of fasting has been recognized and applied from ancient times. Plutarch, the famous biographer (circa A.D. 46-120) said: 'Instead of using medicine, fast a day.'

In an age of pressure, when the breakdown of mind or body, even among professing Christians, is becoming all too familiar, the physical value of God's choosing becomes a matter of some importance. Here is a divine provision for health and healing, for renewal of mind and body, that we must further consider.

Beloved, I pray that . . . you may be in health.

--3 John 2

Your healing shall spring up speedily.

--Isaiah 58:8

Fasting is provided to help us mantain or restore balance and perspective in Kingdom living.

Paul C. Bragg

20

FASTING TO KEEP ARTERIES YOUNG

We are shocked when we hear of the number of people who are killed or injured on the highways in the United States. Some fifty thousand people are killed each year and several million are so seriously injured that they carry the scars for the rest of their lives. We are shocked when we hear of an airplane crashing and killing all the passengers aboard. We are shocked when we see statistics the people who are killed in wars and in police operations all over the world. But the most shocking fact of all is that every second of the entire 24 hours, someone is dying of a heart attack. One out of two all deaths are due to some form of heart trouble. Heart trouble is rightly called the scourge of western civilization. The National Office of Vital Statistics reported in 1973 that almost 1,978,260 deaths in that year were caused by heart and artery trouble. Heart trouble has now reached the epidemic stage.

This enemy of mankind does not select only the older people, but heart trouble of all types is increasing rapidly in young people, also. To give conclusive proof of this statement, an autopsy was performed on 300 men in the armed services who died during the Korean conflict. The autopsy revealed that 77.7% of these young men between 18 and 25 showed deterioration and degeneration of the arteries, particularly of the arteries of the heart.

Diseases of the heart do not build up rapidly. It takes a long time to harden and block an artery and there are many contributing causes ... tobacco, alcohol, excessive eating of saturated fats found in meats, eggs and dairy products, and hydrogenated oils and fats. Another contributing factor that degenerates the arteries is lack of exercise. Frequently, blockage in the arteries is built up to the danger point while the victim is totally unaware of the dangerous situation. It is possible for a person to have arteries half-blocked all over his body without the least sensation that anything is wrong. Even the best doctors, after using all the modern methods of diagnosis, may give him a clean bill of health. The substances that are responsible for the blockage and obstruction of the arteries are cholesterol, fats, and fibrous tissues. As the blockage builds up little by little, the inner passage of the arteries becomes so narrow that enough blood cannot flow through to properly nourish the powerful heart muscle. Coronary occlusion is caused when this serious narrowing of the arteries occurs.

So, you can plainly see that the degeneration of the arteries begins early in life, slowly building up to obstruction and blockage. Then, one fine morning, someone gets up as usual to start the day's activities and suddenly, in the blink of an eye, he either dies abruptly of a heart attack or must live with a very serious chronic condition after the attack.

Constant vigilance must be maintained if the arteries are to be kept free of blockage and obstruction of substances that can cause a heart attack. The heart arteries are small; the largest no wider than a thin soda straw. In the average person who eats the average diet of today, the blockage grows silently, insidiously, and when the blood can no longer flow freely through the great arteries, disaster strikes.

Most people wait until something happens to their arteries before they do anything about it. Because no pains are evident, they continue to eat the bad food, and live with the bad habits that degenerate the arteries.

YOU ARE AS OLD AS YOUR ARTERIES

Again let me repeat the statement - we are all as old as our arteries. Remember that artery-blockage starts even in the very young and slowly builds up until around 55 years of age, when most heart disasters take place.

I want it definitely understood that I do not believe that fasting is a cure for heart trouble. Fasting is a preventive health measure, because, as I have continually stated in this manuscript, fasting is a cleanser of internal impurities. This is exactly how we want to help our arteries - to keep them clean and free of substances that prevent the free flow of blood into the heart and through the entire arterial system.

We have, in the final analysis, a human pipe system that carries our precious five quarts of blood through the entire circulatory system. Our blood circulation must be constantly moving, rhythmically and steadily. For instance, if the flow of blood into the brain is stopped for a fraction of a minute, we could suffer a massive stroke. If it happens in the eye, hemorrhaging can occur that may blind us. The arteries must remain open so the blood will flow to every square inch of the entire body.

Today you will find men and women in their 70's, 80's, and even 90's who have clear, clean, unobstructed, elastic, flexible arteries. Regardless of their calendar years, they are young because their arteries have not degenerated to become obstructed and unflexible. These are the most fortunate people in the world, because if all the organs of their bodies are free from obstruction and toxic materials, there is no reason why these ageless people cannot live for many, many years. In the Bible, we read

that before the great flood, people lived as long as 900 years.
We laugh this off by saying that these people measured their
years in an entirely different way than we do, but how can we be
sure of that? It is quite possible that these people knew how to
eat and live to keep the arteries in perfect working order.
Health is an orderly, harmonious functioning of the body, and this
state of harmony continues as long as the arteries do their work
effectively.

When we speak of people being old, we can only mean one thing -
that they did not know how to eat and live to keep the arteries
unobstructed and elastic. When these damaged arteries are not
doing their work correctly, the blood is not getting into the
brain, and people become senile, forgetful, and often degenerate
to a second childhood. They are dying a slow death because the
blood is not nourishing the brain.

When we fast for a 24-hour period, a 36-hour period, or from
3- to 10-days, all the Vital Power in the body is used for internal purification, and that also means purification of the arteries
in the body. That is why many times after a 10-day fast, there
will be a feeling of lightness in the body, the mind will become
keener and more alert, and the memory will improve. The
craving for physical activity will become intense. Because of
the lightness that comes over the body, I feel that fasting helps
to keep our arteries clean, elastic, and youthful.

I must reiterate the importance of a thorough check of the urine.
During the 10-day fast, it is bottled each morning and saved for
future observation. The faster will note a tremendous amount
of heavy foreign substances that have been eliminated from the
body, particularly, the heavy mucus condition that appears in
the urine.

In my opinion, we can add years to our hearts with a systematic
program of fasting, coupled with a program of natural food which
reduces the waxy substance that forms in the arteries. I believe
we must think of our arteries as the key to life if we want to
win the greatest battle we will ever face - that of staying alive
on this earth. When you stuff yourself on fatty meals, day
after day, you are bound to accumulate poisons and osbstruc-
tions. Retribution is bound to come. The body requires only a
very small amount of fat every day, yet we are the greatest
consumers of fat in the world, and we consequently lead the
world in diseases of the heart and the arteries.

This is one reason that I believe in the no-breakfast plan. I
have known many young, healthy, brilliant men and women who
made it a habit every morning to eat a so-called hearty breakfast of ham and eggs, or bacon and eggs, buttered toast, fried

potatoes, and coffee loaded with cream. I also know that many of these supposedly healthy people were stricken with heart attacks that either killed them or made them invalids for the rest of their lives. You cannot eat any food simply because you think it agrees with you, and you won't make this mistake if you know something about the physiology of the body and about nutrition. Eating is a science, which means more than tickling the palate. Eating is a serious function, particularly if you want to keep your arteries clean, unobstructed, and unblocked.

Before you go on the program that I have outlined in this book, get a thorough physical examination by a good heart doctor, and let him acquaint you with the condition of your arteries and heart. Know your blood pressures, know your pulse, and then follow this system of living for a year. Then return to your doctor and let him examine you again. I believe that your doctor will say that you have created a miracle in your body in one short year. Again, let me repeat that you are only as young as your arteries. Your arteries tell your age, not your birthdays.

THE HEART AND CIRCULATORY SYSTEM

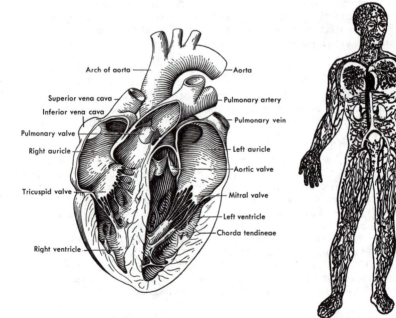

The heart is really a double pump, each side composed of two chambers, an auricle and a ventricle.

Circulatory system. Showing arteries and veins.

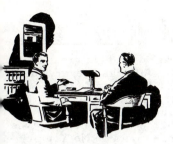

YOU HAVE
NINE DOCTORS
AT YOUR COMMAND

Nature's nine physicians are ready to help you attain radiant, glorious health. They are all specialists in their particular field of health-building. They have had years and years of experience with thousands upon thousands of people. Their cumulative record is one hundred percent perfect. They have never failed a patient ... patients have failed them, turned their backs on them, and ignored them. But they are kind and understanding, and no matter how many times patients have failed them, they still stand ready to render perfect professional service. They have but one prescription and that is elixir of LIFE.

They are the kindest doctors in the whole universe. They are anxious and willing to help everyone who comes to them for Health ... their professional services are available to all — the young, the old, the rich, and the poor. They give no operations ... except bloodless ones. They give no drugs ... not even the latest "Wonder" drugs.

You are all familiar with these nine doctors ... and from time to time many of you have needed their services and called upon them. But, from this day on, I want you to call on these nine doctors frequently ... they are so anxious to Help You Help Yourself to Health, Long Life, and that extra-special physical condition known as "AGELESSNESS"! That is the Highest Health you can have ... and I DO want you to have the finest.

These wonderful physicians will never, ever fail you. They not only want to be your personal physicians, but they want to be your friends. It gives me a most secure feeling that I have, at my command every day, the world's great physicians.

Now, it is my pleasure to give you a personal introduction to each one of these physicians, and, from this day on, feel free to call upon them. First, I want you to meet the Daddy of them all, the most eminent, the most powerful, the great Healer, the giver of life to everything on the face of this earth. It is my pleasure to introduce to you the nine doctors.

Doctor Sunshine's specialty is heliotheraphy, and his great prescription is solar energy. Each tiny blade of grass, every vine, tree, bush, flower, fruit, and vegetable draws its life from solar energy. All living things on earth depend on solar energy for their very existence. This earth would be a barren, frigid place if it were not for the magic rays of the sun. The sun gives us light, and were it not for LIGHT, there would be No You or Me. The earth would be in everlasting darkness. Human Beings were never meant to have pale skins, not even the fair northern races. Man's skin should be tanned by sun and air, and should take on a darker pigment according to his original type. It has been found that under constant sun even red-headed people will tan. Pigmentation is a sign that solar energy has been transformed into human energy. Man can only gain health, vitality, and happiness in the bright, brilliant rays of the sun. The people who are indoors too long have a sallow ghastly-looking skin. That is why so many women hide their yellow, sun-starved skins with makeup.

The person who is starved of the vital rays of the sun has a half dead look. He is actually dying for the want of solar energy. Weak, ailing, anemic people are all sun-starved, and in my opinion, many people are sick simply because they too are starving for sunshine.

The rays of the sun are powerful germicides. As the skin imbibes more of these rays, it stores up enormous amounts of this germ-killing energy. The sun provides one of the finest remedies for the nervous person, who is filled with anxiety, worry, frustration, stresses, and strains. When these tense people lie in the sunshine, its powerful rays give them what the nerves and body are crying out for, and that is relaxation. Sunshine is a tonic, a stimulant and above all, the GREAT HEALER! As you bask in the warm sunshine, millions of nerve endings absorb the solar energy and transform it to the nervous system of the body.

Make this experiment determine the value of sunshine in the matter of life and death. Find a beautiful lawn, where the grass is like a green carpet... Cover up a small space of that beautiful lawn with a small piece of wood or a piece of metal. Day by day you will notice that the beautiful grass that is full of plant blood, Chlorophyll, will start to fade and turns a sickly yellow. Then the tragedy happens - it withers and dies - death by sun starvation.

The same thing happens in your body without the life-giving rays of the sun, and when you fail to eat an abundance of sun-cooked foods such as ripe fruits, and vegetables.

We must have the direct rays of the sun on our bodies and we must eat at least 50 percent of food that has been ripened by the sun's rays. When we eat fresh fruits and vegetables, we absorb blood of the plant, the rich, nourishing Chlorophyll. Chlorophyll is the solar energy that the plant has absorbed from the sun, the richest and most nourishing food you can put into your body. "Chlorophyll is liquid sunshine". Green plants alone possess the secret of how to capture this powerful solar energy and pass it on to man and every other living creature. When you put sunshine on the outside of your body, and eat 50 percent raw fruits and vegetables in your daily diet, you are going to fairly glow with radiant health.

But these too-powerful, natural medicines must be taken in very small doses at the beginning, because your sun-starved body cannot absorb too great an amount at first.

When you take your first sun bath, start with short time periods until you can condition your body to take more and more. The best time for a beginner to start taking sun baths is in the early morning sunshine... five to ten minutes on the nude body is sufficient at first. Or you may sunbathe in the late afternoon sunshine. The best rays of the sun are in the early morning... these have the cooling rays. Between 11 to 3 we have the hot burning rays of the sun.

The same caution should be taken in eating sun-ripened foods... the raw fruits and vegetables. The average person who has been eating mainly cooked foods will find that... if suddenly great amounts of raw fruit and vegetables are put into the body they can cause a reaction. It is wiser to gradually add more and more sun-cooked foods to the diet. Overdoses of solar energy, both outside the body and in the body, are not good. In exposure to the sun, it is quite necessary to use good judgment and proceed with caution. Here, I must add a personal touch... At 16 years of age I had been sentenced to death with deadly tuberculosis. The greatest doctors in the United States declared me "Hopeless - Incurable!" But, by the Grace of God, I was led to Dr. August Rollier of Leysen, Switzerland, the greatest living authority on Heliotheraphy - (Sun Cure). High in the Alps, Dr. Rollier exposed my sick, wasting body to the healing rays of the sun and fed me an abundance of sun-cooked foods. And Presto! A miracle happened. In two short years I was transformed from my death-bed to a vitally strong young man... and today at 85 years young as I write this, I am still a powerful and healthy man. Through all of these years, I have kept the pigmentation of the sun's rays continually in my body. I regained my health through "Dr. Healing Sunshine"... he saved my life... and that is why I am a sun worshiper of God's own precious sunshine. That is why I make my home in California, the great sunshine state, (except Los Angeles where the sickening smog has replaced the sunshine). I have a cabin high in the Santa Monica mountains so that I may get the benefit of the mountain sunshine. I have a modest home in the California Desert, where the sun shines 354 days a year. I am a great beach boy...I spend long hours, both in winter and summer, on the great beaches of the world...Hawaii, Florida, at Cannes in France, on the sun-drenched islands of the Aegean Sea...Rhodes...Crete and Capri. Seek the sun and Health will come by leaps and bounds.

★ ★ ★ ★ ★

Actress Cloris Leachman, an ardent health follower — who sparkles with health, hates smoking, coffee, hard booze and sugar and meat, and one of her solutions to the problems of the body is to fast. "Fasting is simply wonderful. I can do practically anything. It is a miracle cure. It cured my asthma."

E. M. Forster, one of Britain's literary immortals, observed that food is one of the five main facts of life, "a link between the known and the forgotten." It was a marvel to him that we can go on "day after day putting an assortment of objects into a hole in our faces without becoming surprised or bored."

In the course of a year the average adult eats 120 pounds of sugar, 53 pounds of fats, 100 pounds of white flour, 14 pounds of white rice, 25 pounds of potatoes, and five pounds of ice cream.

There can be no arguing that many mouths function as litter baskets and garbage dumps.

"A full stomach does not like to think."

Old German Proverb

"Privation of food at first brings a sensation of hunger, occasionally some nervous stimulation . . . but it also determines certain hidden phenomena which are more important. The sugar of the liver and the fat of the subcutaneous deposits are mobilized, and also the proteins of the muscles and glands. All the organs sacrifice their own substances in order to maintain blood, heart, and brain in a normal condition. Fasting purifies and profoundly modifies our tissues."

—Dr. Alexis Carrel
Nobel Prize-winner/*Man, the Unknown*

He fasted forty days and forty nights, and afterward he was hungry.
--Matthew 4:2

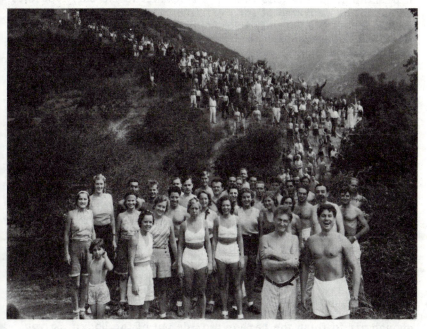

A Thousand Happy Hikers Enjoying Exercise and Fresh Air on The Trail to Mt. Hollywood, California. Summer, 1932. Bernarr Macfadden, Left - Father and Founder of the Physical Culture Movement and Pioneer Physical Culture Magazine and Paul C. Bragg, right - Life Extension Specialist - enjoyed leading Health and Fitness Seminars across the United States.

Dr. Fresh Air is a specialist, and his greatest prescription is "The Breath of God's Pure Fresh Air."

The first thing we do when we are born is to take a long, deep breath and the last thing we do is take a last gasp, before we stop breathing. Between birth and death, life is completely maintained by breathing.

Dr. Fresh Air wants you to have a long active life and he feels, as a specialist, that if you follow his simple instructions of breathing deeply, always being conscious that with every breath you take, you are bringing into your body the breath of God, the life-giving oxygen.

People who fail to obey the doctor's orders about getting plenty of fresh air day and night, invite some extremely severe complications. Let us examine very closely the function of breathing. First it is invisible food...it is the only food that we cannot be deprived of for over five to seven minutes or death will take us. We not only take from the air the life-giving oxygen that is so necessary to every cell in our bodies, but when we breathe oxygen, it is carried by the blood to the lungs and there a great miracle takes place. The life-giving oxygen is exchanged for deadly carbon dioxide in which form the deadly toxins of the body are being released. In other words, in the process of living, we create toxic poisons. They are collected by the blood, and when the blood brings carbon dioxide to the lungs, it is expelled as the new life-giving oxygen enters. In the process of metabolism in the building up and tearing down of the cells of the body, carbon dioxide poison is constantly burned up in the very process of living.

If a person does not get enough fresh air, or if he is a shallow breather, and the intake of oxygen does not equal the outgo of carbon dioxide, we are encouraging carbon dioxide toxic poison to build within the structure of the body. This can result in very serious physical problems, because the retained carbon dioxide can be concentrated in some other part of the body and cause intense physical suffering.

Enervation, or the lack of nerve energy, can lower the Vital Force so much that the great bellows, the lungs, cannot pump in enough air to flush the carbon dioxide out of the body. So you see how important it is that you not only breathe fresh air, but you should be always conscious of the fact that you must breathe deeply.

I believe we are air machines. I believe that oxygen not only purifies our body, but is also one of the great energizers of the human body. We are air-pressure machines. We live at the bottom of an atmospheric ocean approximately 70 miles deep. This air pressure is 14 pounds per square inch. Between the inhalation and the exhalation of a breath, a vacuum is formed. As long as we continue to have this rhythmical intake and outgo of oxygen, we will live. We know that we can go without food for 30 days or more and still survive, but as I have stated, we can only go without air for a very few minutes, so air is one of the important energizers of the human body. The more deeply you breathe pure air, the better your chances are for extending your years on this earth.

For over 70 years, I have done extensive research on long-lived people and I find one common denominator among all of them. They are deep breathers. I have found that the deeper, therefore fewer breaths a person takes in one minute, the longer they live, and the rapid breathers are the short-lived people. This is also true in the animal world. Rabbits, guinea pigs, and all k is of rodents are rapid breathers, taking many deep breaths every minute. They are the shortest-lived breathing creatures on the face of the earth. For years I have made it a practice when I first get up in the morning to take long, slow, deep breaths. And all during my waking hours, I try to take periods where I breathe long, full deep breaths.

INDIA HOLY MEN PRACTICE DEEP, SLOW BREATHING

In my expeditions into India, I found holy men in secluded re- treats who had devoted their lives to building a physically power- ful body as an instrument for high spiritual advancement. They spend many hours daily in the practice of rhythmic, long, slow deep breaths. These holy men of India were utterly fantastic, physically, because the deep breathing of fresh air kept their skin and muscle-tone ageless. I met a holy man in the foothills of the Himalaya Mountains, who told me that he was, at that time, 126 years old. This man had no reason to lie to me, because his whole life was spent in getting closer to God. It was he who taught me the system which I teach all over the world, known as "Super Brain-Breathing". I do not have sufficient space in this book to go into detail about the full program that this holy man taught me, but you may write for this manuscript "Super Brain Breathing" and my other health books listed on the back of this book.

To go further in describing this holy man physically, he had per- fect vision, and he had a beautiful head of hair with not one gray hair in it. He had all his teeth, and he had the endurance and stamina of an athlete. He spoke seven languages fluently...he was one of the most amazing men that I have ever met in my life, and when I asked him to what circumstance he owed his great strength, and mentality, his answer was, "I have made a long life practice of breathing deeply and practicing faithfully all of my breathing exercises daily."

As a man, I do not like to guess the age of any woman, but while I was on this trip to India, I met a woman, whose age I guessed as about 50. I was amazed when she told me she was 86. She was a beautiful woman with no sign of deterioration, and I asked her the secret of her beauty and her agelessness and again I got the same answer I did from the holy man - this beautiful woman was conscious of the importance of deep breathing.

You have noticed children running and playing, jumping rope, rollerskating, and bicycling. While they are doing these activi- ties, they are breathing in large amounts of oxygen, and that is what we must keep in mind. We must keep active. We must take long, brisk walks. I realize that we live in an air-polluted world today, but that is all the more reason that we should cul- tivate the habit of deep breathing. When I find people living

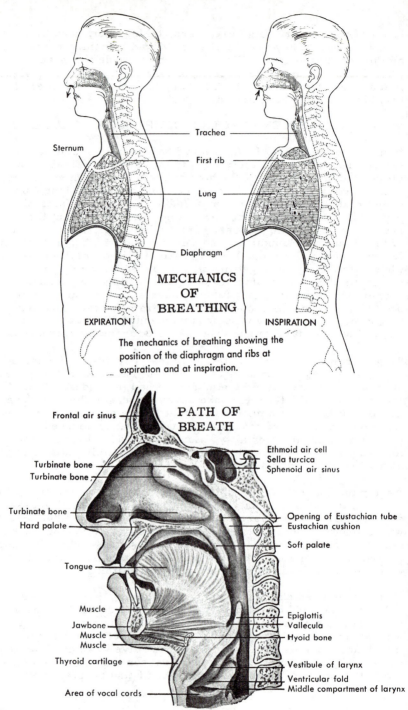

Trachea

Sternum

First rib

Lung

Diaphragm

MECHANICS OF BREATHING

EXPIRATION

INSPIRATION

The mechanics of breathing showing the position of the diaphragm and ribs at expiration and at inspiration.

PATH OF BREATH

Frontal air sinus

Ethmoid air cell
Sella turcica
Sphenoid air sinus

Turbinate bone
Turbinate bone

Turbinate bone
Hard palate

Opening of Eustachian tube
Eustachian cushion

Soft palate

Tongue

Muscle
Jawbone
Muscle
Muscle

Epiglottis
Vallecula
Hyoid bone

Thyroid cartilage

Vestibule of larynx

Area of vocal cords

Ventricular fold
Middle compartment of larynx

sedentary lives, no longer getting vigorous exercise, I know that they are shortening their lives.

DEEP BREATHING SECRET OF ENDURANCE AND STAMINA

I had a friend for many years named Amos Stagg, the famous football and athletic coach. Mr. Stagg lived to be over 100 years of age. I asked him his secret of long life and his answer was "I have the greater part of my life indulged in running and other vigorous exercise that forced large amounts of oxygen into my body."

I had a friend in New York, James Hocking, who was one of the greatest long distance walking champions this country has ever had. I asked Mr. Hocking, on his hundredth birthday, the secret of his long, active life and super-health. His answer was "I have always walked vigorously and breathed deeply".

So you see, oxygen is a detoxifier. It is like fasting...it removes poisons from the body.

I not only practice deep breathing personally, but I also believe that people should expose their bodies to a free current of moving air. Air baths are important to good health. You should sleep with your windows wide open with a cross ventilation of air moving across you as you sleep. I find that I sleep better, and have a deeper night's rest, if I don't wear sleeping garments of any kind. Under the covers it is warm and when we pile on extra sleeping garments, we shut off the skin from its supply of oxygen. You must compensate for your hours of sitting down because it is then that your breathing slows down. So if your occupation requires a lot of sitting, you should compensate with outdoor walking and physical activities.

You will find that you can solve most of your problems on a brisk 2- or 3-mile hike. Whenever I have a problem to solve, I always take a long brisk walk in the fresh air, and by the time I have finished the walk, I have solved my problems. I believe that after the evening meal, everyone should make a practice of taking a 2-mile walk (even if it has to be up and down your driveway.) Today we are a race of sitters. We sit at our desks, at the movies, concerts, and sit watching athletics and television. We are air-starved, we are oxygen-starved. We cannot get carbon dioxide out of our bodies, and so we are full of aches, pains, and prone to premature aging. This is all because we are too lazy, too indifferent about being active, vigorous people. On any city street, you can see nothing but pale, ghastly people, unhealthy and exhausted, all because of air-starvation. That is

why it is so important to fast, because then you clean some of
this concentrated, stored carbon dioxide that failed to leave your
body by deep breathing.

So when you are fasting, whether it is day or night, and if you
have the energy, take a walk, even if it is a short one. Between
fasting, make it a part of your life to be an active person. That
does not mean house-walks, it means getting out in the fresh air
and hiking, or running, or swimming, or dancing. You must
not allow carbon dioxide to pile up in your body, it can only bring
serious consequences. So, along with your fasting program,
make it a point every day of your life to have a vigorous 2-mile
walk and, during that walk, breathe deeply. Every time you
think of it during your waking hours, take long, slow, deep
breaths. Remember what I told you, the fewer long, slow, deep
breaths you take, the longer you will live, and when you combine
deep breathing with fasting, you are adding years to your life.
You are building energy and vitality. You are going to break
free of many miseries with fasting and deep breathing, so remind
yourself every day that Doctor Fresh Air is your constant friend.

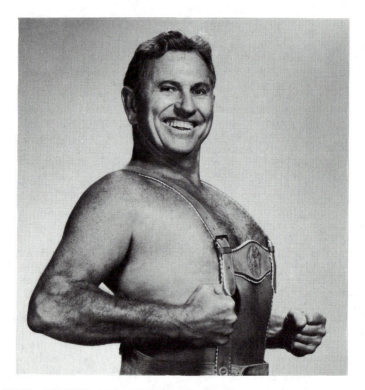

CLEAN, FRESH AIR BUILT BRAGG A POWERFUL BODY

23

DOCTOR PURE WATER

Dr. Pure Water is a fine physician and a splendid friend. I have told you in another part of this manuscript the importance of drinking distilled water. I will not elaborate on that here. Water makes up about 70 percent of your body so you need a continuous replacement to keep the water level normal. As you add more raw fruit and vegetables to your diet, you will add a greater intake of natural distilled water. Dr. Pure Water is a friend, and you may enjoy many pleasant hours using the various gains that water gives you. A good warm bath is a tonic and a relaxer which soothes irritated nerves and quiets emotions. Every day of the year in the United States, people enjoy water at the sea shore, in lakes, rivers, streams, and swimming pools. Swimming is one of the best exercises anyone can take. It puts no strain on the human body or the heart. Make it a point to swim as often as you can. If you can't swim, go to a professional who can teach you how to swim. You will never regret it, because it is one of the most relaxing, and yet, exhilarating of exercises. It can be enjoyed regardless of your age. Don't fear it — learn to love it.

Water has been used as a treatment for man's miseries since the very beginning of time and in my travels all over the world, I have found, as a Physical Therapist, many types of water treatments. It has been proven that the ancient civilizations of the Egyptians, the Assyrians, Hebrews, Persians, Greeks, Hindus, Chinese, and many other races, including the American Indians, have used all forms of water treatment for the relief of human ailments. Hippocrates, the father of medicine, 400 years before the birth of Christ on the island of Coo in the Aegean Sea, developed a complete system of water treatments. His records state that a cold bath followed by a hot bath and then followed by friction improve the circulation. We cannot surmount that natural philosophy today. The cold, then hot bath with a coarse friction rub with a towel, is one of the best circulation builders known to man.

I have visited practically all the great Health Spas in the world. I have a home in Desert Hot Springs, California so I may enjoy the healing waters of this "Spa City". It is called the healthiest city in the United States. It is located directly on the Andreas fault where many earthquakes originate. Under this fault at Desert Hot Springs, there is a great river of red-hot, mineral water. Wells are piped down to the river, and the hot mineral water is brought to the spas. People from all over the world come to Desert Hot Springs to bathe in the soothing, hot mineral water. I do not regard hot water as a cure for any human ailment, but I believe that hot water, particularly at 104°, is a purifier and a detoxifier and an exhilirator of circulation. This is why I recommend a hot Epsom Salt bath every few weeks as a purifier, detoxifier, and relaxer. It is taken in water anywhere from 98° to 104°. You should remain in this bath from 5 to 10 minutes, and no more. Along with a fasting program, the every two week hot Epsom salt bath can be a very important part of your program of natural living, but never take your hot Epsom bath during your fasting time. **Steam distilled water is the best to use.**

Clean, pure water inside and outside is one of Nature's wonderful ways of building a healthy body.

WATER — MORE IMPORTANT THAN FOOD

More than one-half of the human body is water. The bones in you your body are even one-third water. To lose a tenth of your body's water supply is dangerous, and to lose a fifth can be fatal. Losing lesser amounts disturbs body functions and impairs chemical and physical processes necessary to good health. Yet, the body itself, can take lots of punishment — half your proteins can be lost and almost all of your fat and glycogen without causin death. Only that important fifty-five percent of your body — water — requires that it be kept at a consistently high level.

A practical example of the body's demand for water can be drawn from mountain climbing histories. In the assault on the Himalayas, men working and climbing in high altitudes cut down on the weight they carried in an attempt to conserve body energy. None were notably successful until the team conquering Mount Everest scientifically considered the effect of the altitude in relation to bodily water metabolism. These men increased their fuel load in order to melt snow and ice into water. They were assured of an average of six pints per day per man, much more than previous teams had considered as adequate rations. While water was not the sole contributing factor to their success, it was recognized as helping prevent the fatigue experienced by former teams during their final assaults.

We, ourselves, may not need water for anything as demanding as climbing the Himalayas, but this serves as an example of how important water — or the lack of water — in our diets can be.

★ ★ ★ ★ ★

What sculpture is to a block of marble, education is to the soul.

- Addison, The Spectator

In the 1959 Yearbook of Agriculture, United States Department of Agriculture, on page 168, Dr. Olaf Mickelson states:

Next to oxygen, water is the most important factor for survival of man and animals. A person can do without food for 5 weeks or more, but without water he can survive for only a few days.

Again, in a report prepared for Office of Civil Defense Mobilization, Western Regional Research Laboratory, USDA, Albany, California by R. L. Olson, Vern F. Kaufman and Eleanor C. Taylor say:

Food is probably not necessary for bare survival for healthy people for two weeks. Most of the population could live if nothing but adequate water were available.

HOW OUR BODY USES WATER

Almost every fluid connected with life and living things is based on water. Protoplasm cannot exist without water. Nor can a blade of grass, or a cactus, or an insect, or a bird or a fish. Dry out a living cell and it will stop working. It must have liquid. Human cells are the very same. Even their food is brought to them via fluid — blood. And there are about ten pounds of blood alone in your body. After food is consumed by cells, the waste is washed away in a water-based liquid called urine. Even oxygen cannot be absorbed by your lungs except through a moist surface. The same is true of the waste by-product of oxygen, carbon dioxide.

To quote W. B. Cannon,

"Water is the vehicle for food materials absorbed from the digestive canal; it is the medium in which chemical changes take place that underlie most of our obvious activities; it is essential in the regulation of body temperature, and it plays an important part in mechanical services such as the lubrication ... of joint surfaces ... "

WATER AND DIGESTION

Food can't be digested without water. There is an actual chemical process that goes on in your body that's known as "hydrolysis." It involves changing proteins, starches and fats into foods that various cells require in order to work properly. But water is also necessary to stimulate gastric glands in the stomach. In the intestines, it helps facilitate the absorption of solids — and the excretion of wastes.

Let's take a look at how water is important to digestion by starting with the intake of food at the mouth. Here, the 99-1/2% water fluid known as saliva begins the digestion of carbohydrates. The gastric juices we've mentioned are 90% water and they work on the food passed to the stomach. The food, now fairly liquid, is passed to the duodenum, or upper section of the small intestine where enzymes, liver secretions and pancreas (90% water) finish digestion of food.

Food is passed on through the small and large intestines and is absorbed through intestinal walls in a watery state. The largest portion of the absorption of the water itself occurs in the colon. When not absorbed, diarrhea results. Water not absorbed is passed as waste, a dangerous situation in infants who, because of their size, have only a small supply of water. This can result in dehydration, bad digestion and even death.

Somewhere between seven and eleven quarts of water are needed just for proper digestion. Breaking this down, it comes to three pints of saliva, a couple of quarts of gastric juice, plus an equivalent amount as bile and other glandular and intestinal secretions. Fortunately, the body is thrifty and most of this is absorbed again and re-used.

Its first job after being absorbed is to transfer the new digested foods to the cells through the blood stream, the blood cells themselves using and re-using the water in their own process of living.

WATER AND WASTE

While water plays an important role in the excretion of waste through the intestine, most of it is re-absorbed and doesn't leave the body. But the other forms of soluble waste rely on water, too. The kidneys (and bladder), skin and lungs all depend on water to rid themselves of poisons and excretions.

The lung-wall is comprised of tiny air sacs that, in order to function in the intake of oxygen and the expulsion of carbon dioxide, must be moist. The linings of the nose, throat, trachea and bronchial tubes are also always moist — or should be. Because of all this contact with air, the body loses about a pint of water every day solely through exhalation. When the air is very dry, more is lost. Many people replace this moisture by using a vaporizer in their homes.

Water lost through the skin can amount to large quantities, but here water is used not only as a vehicle for waste, but for other purposes and is discussed elsewhere in this book.

Kidneys use water rapidly, but the amount they use depends on the amount of fluid you drink. For every quart of water passed through the kidneys, one and a half ounces of waste are carried in it. This is normal, but water (as urine) never falls below a level of a little more than half a pint. Kidneys never stop working and constantly demand water, even when none is available. The body is forced to supply it through dehydration as long as there is life.

All this occurs without any chemical transformation of the water. It might be named for its contents, but it carries them is solution. The water remains water.

BLOOD AND WATER

Sure, blood is thicker than water. But only by about 10%. Blood plasma is 90% water and permits it to circulate through the body freely. It carries all sorts of foods and gases, inorganic salts and products, wastes and items needed for body functions, activity and growth.

Everything used by body cells is transported by plasma, including the material the cell is made from. Anything made by these same cells needed in other parts of the body — or to be excreted — is carried by the same plasma. Yet, plasma remains fairly identical in composition at all times at all places in the body. As it absorbs foods and fuels from the digestive and respiratory processes, it has the same foods and fuels taken from it by body tissues — including the kidneys and lungs. A balance is always maintained, and water (the proper intake) is important.

WATER KEEPS YOU COOL

Automobiles have water in their radiators to help cool their engines. It's much the same with the human body. The reason is that water absorbs heat readily. In living organisms, where constant internal temperatures are often vital, water acts as a super-efficient coolant. The human body has a constant temperature level. Measured orally, this is 98.6°F. And, it shouldn't vary much despite the climate or temperature surrounding the body.

This internal temperature is controlled by external skin evaporation to a large degree. Just about a fourth of the heat created in the burning of oxygen and food by the body is thrown off the body by normal perspiration, and by the process of breathing.

But, under exceptionally dry conditions, the body can lose up to a quart an hour through the sweating process alone. Obviously, this water has to be replaced or other functions of the body are imparied. When it's cold, the body can actually cease perspiring and water is further withdrawn into the tissues. The evaporation of water from skin surfaces results in cooling — air-conditioning. It's related to fever. When you sweat and feel hot, perhaps you have a temperature. When your skin is dry and you feel chills, perhaps body temperature has dipped. Signs of illness.

And, of course, in humid weather, evaporation is more difficult. So we feel hotter though we're sweating. Our body is having a harder time cooling off, and ends up working harder to keep it cool.

Researchers have found the average man, doing nothing, on a normally humid day will lose about twenty-three ounces of fluid via lungs and skin per day. A long-distance runner, on the other hand, has lost as much as eight pounds.

Football players have lost almost fourteen pounds of water alone in about an hour's time. Because the body is more than one-half water, and because excretory processes depend so much on water, water is easy to lose and many so-called diets are often based on lower water consumption or higher water loss. This can be very dangerous, especially if protracted over a period of time. Tired ness is one of the first signs of water deficiency. It should be heeded. Take a drink.

WATER IS A LUBRICANT

The body, in its own way, is greased and oiled automatically. The basic lubricant is water. It permits organs to slide against each other — such as when you bend down. It helps bones slip in their joints. You couldn't bend a knee or elbow without it. Also, it acts as a shock absorbing agent to ward off injury from blows. Applied hydraulically to various parts of the body, it is used to build and hold pressures. The eyeball is a good example of this function of water.

Muscle tone cannot be kept without adequate water, for the muscles are three-fourths water. This is another reason why fatigue hits the dehydrated body.

THREE SOURCES FOR WATER

Your body has to come by its water somehow. The first way is obvious. You drink it — or a fluid containing water such a fruit juice, coffee, soup, beverages, and the like. Regular foods are sources of water supply, too. Don't forget, your own body is about 70% water — so little wonder that steak should be about 60% water. An egg is more than two-thirds water. A peach is almost all water — 90%. Something as dry as a hard roll even is a fourth water.

The third, important source is metabolism. This water is called metabolic water and it's made by the body from raw materials taken into the body. In other words, it's a chemically made water. It happens when cells convert ingested food to cellular food. A perfect example of this type of water production is that water-factory known as the camel. Now, the camel doesn't store water. It stores fat in the hump on its back. It also eats carbohydrates. In using these foods, the camel creates a great deal of water as a by-product — and uses the water in its body chemistry just as if it had drunk the water! Some insects are able to do this, too, even though they eat exceptionally dry, low-water-content foods.

While the average man only consumes about two and a half quarts of water a day by eating and drinking, he uses up a full two and three fourths quarts. (4.922 grams vs. 5.210 grams) His production of metabolic water is the difference.

BODY THIRST

When the body hasn't enough water, it reacts. First, the secretions of glands are drastically cut. Saliva dries up, membranes dry out. We're thirsty. We've been signaled quickly that a drink of water is imperative. After losing more than a little water without replenishing the supply, other symptoms develop. Headaches, nerves, inability to concentrate, digestion problems, lack of hunger are some of these. Water quickly alleviates these symptoms. American soldiers in the artic experienced personality problems when forced into low-water rations because of the lack of fuel. As mentioned elsewhere, to be deprived of water for just a few days can invite death. It is needed continuously.

THE VINEGAR AND WATER COCKTAIL AIDS
IN KEEPING THE URINE ACID

The vinegar and water cocktail taken the first thing in the morning aids in keeping the urine in an acid condition. Acid is the natural condition of the urine. This shows the kidneys are doing their duties efficiently slushing out the body poisons. The cocktail consists of a 6 oz. glass of distilled water and two teaspoons of raw natural unpasterurized and unfiltered vinegar that has been aged in wood. (Many brands of this natural vinegar are sold in Health Food Stores.)

Go to any good drug store and purchase Squibb-Nitrazine paper. Dip a small piece of this paper in your urine sample immediately. There is a chart on the nitrazine paper container for you to compare the urine. If it is yellow your urine is normal, that means it is acid. The chart will give you truthful answer.
Apples, grapes, cranberries, strawberries, cherries and raspberries will aid in keeping your urine the normal acid.

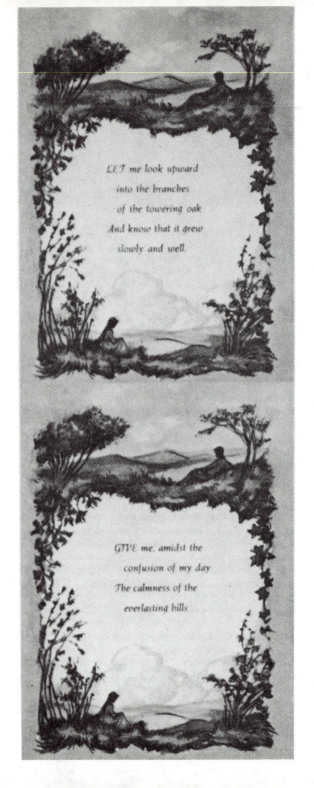

*LET me look upward
into the branches
of the towering oak
And know that it grew
slowly and well.*

*GIVE me, amidst the
confusion of my day
The calmness of the
everlasting hills . . .*

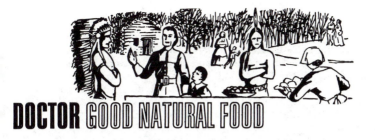

24

DOCTOR GOOD NATURAL FOOD

Your body is the most gloriously accurate instrument in this universe. Given the correct fuel, pure air, exercise, sunshine and keeping it internally clean by fasting, your body will last indefinitely and function perfectly.

A healthy body is an efficient chemical factory. Given the correct raw materials, it should be capable, except for accidents, of developing strong tissues and good resistance against most bacteria, viruses, and other environmental impacts.

It is the only fine machine I know that contains its own repair shop and can work wonders if you give it the proper tools. It is constantly working for you. Its cells are being destroyed and renewed every second. Biologically, it has no age limit, and, in fact there is no biological reason for man to grow old at all.

The body has the seed of eternal life. Man does not die - he commits slow suicide with his unnatural habits of living.

Scientists tell us that every cell in our body is renewed within eleven months. Then why should anyone speak of being old?

Don't you believe the moth-eaten fallacy that man, as he gets older, must face decrepitude, decay, senility and death.

If people knew what to eat and would eat what they should, Old Father Time would shoulder his scythe and walk off in the other direction.

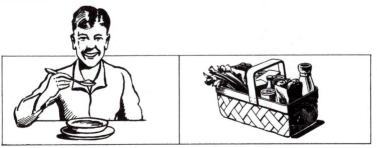

Universally people are suffering from mineral and vitamin starvation. Research shows that thousands of people are victims of malnutrition. The millions of red blood cells in the body are constantly dying and being replaced, some of them being renewed every second. But they cannot be renewed properly without the right substance. The right substance must come from food - good, wholesome, natural food. The person you are today, the person you will be tomorrow, next week, next month, ten years from now, depends on what you eat! You are the sum total of the food you consume. How you look, how you feel, how you carry your years, all of these depend on what you eat!

Every part of your body is made from food - the hair on your head, your eyes, teeth, bones, blood and flesh. Even your expression is formed from what you eat, because the healthy man is a well-fed, happy man.

We often jokingly say "What are we going to feed our faces?" when it is plain that we mean our entire bodies (including our faces) are ready for nourishment.

We can begin anywhere in the body but there is some logic in starting with the skeleton which supports all other tissues. Superficially, our bones are largely mineral matter-mostly calcium and phosphate. One might suppose that once the skeleton is formed, nutrition of the bone stops. This is far from true. With "isotopic tracers", biochemists have found that even in an adult body, minerals are constantly leaving and entering the bones. This means that bones are alive; the situation is dynamic rather than static. Bones contain living bone cells which require not only minerals for building bone, but all the other food nutrients that living cells need in order to maintain themselves.

An emergency need for these cells arises when a bone becomes broken. If these cells had ceased to live and function when the adult skeleton became formed, a broken bone would remain broken for the rest of one's life. When a bone does become broken, nourishment of these bone cells is crucially important, they not only need the minerals required for repairing the damage but the cells themselves need to "eat" and keep well.

These bone cells, like all other cells, can be nourished at various levels of efficiency. This is related to the fact that sometimes bones knit slowly and sometimes rapidly. The rate of healing can be retarded by relatively poor nutrition of the cells that do the repair work; it can be stepped up by improving the nutrition of these cells. Good physicians who treat fracture cases, especially those who are nutrition-minded, take pains to see that every possible measure is taken to promote the finest nutrition possible to build new bone cells.

ENTIRE BODY NEEDS NATURAL NUTRITION

The cells in our skin, including the hair-building cells need continual nourishment; this becomes more evident and compelling when we remember that skin is constantly being worn away and replaced, and hair grows continuously, day and night, year after year.

Those who handle farm animals, pets, or racing animals know that skin and hair-sleekness is an important index of health and well being. If an animal's hair or fur is well nourished and healthy, this is an indication that the other cells of its body are at least fairly well-nourished. Laboratory experience with mammals and fowl shows that many entirely different nutritional deficiencies will cause the skin and hair, or feathers, to become unhealthy and disheveled in appearance.

Nutritionists recognize the appearance of healthy skin and are often able to judge the person's condition on this basis. Several gross vitamin deficiencies in human beings are obvious in the unhealthy appearance of the skin.

That national misery, constipation, is often a manifestation of wrong nutrition of the intestinal tissues. In the intestinal tract, there are many involuntary "smooth" muscles which, when stimulated, cause stomach and intestinal movements. These wave-like motions keep the partially digested food moving along until the residue reaches the large bowel and is eventually eliminated. All the smooth muscles are made up of living cells which must be nourished to a high level of efficiency if the whole process is to proceed with facility. In order to prevent stagnation in the intestinal tract, irritating substances (powerful laxatives) are often used. These stimulate and "drive" the muscle cells, sometimes mercilessly, when usually all that muscle cells need to function efficiently is bulk to work on, coupled with good sound nutrition habits.

The system of arteries, veins, and capillaries which carries blood and nourishment to all parts of the body are not inert pipes; their walls contain indispensable living cells which must be nourished satisfactorily in order to remain alive and well. They do not always stay well, as in the case of so-called hardening of the arteries which results from an unhealthy, "corroded" condition which can certainly be aggravated by improper nutrition.

The center of the circulatory system - the heart, is very much alive and its continual nourishment is crucially important. It pumps blood all over the body, but the heart is a powerful muscle which utilizes a tremendous amount of energy and the heart-muscle cells need to be "fed" a highly nutritious "natural diet", day in and day out. If an artery supplying blood to the heart becomes unhealthy and corroded, it is more likely to be stopped-up by a small blood-clot. In this case, the heart-muscle cells which depend on the artery for sustenance are starved. If the starvation, particularly for oxygen, is extensive and lasts even a fraction of a minute, the victim may die of a coronary heart attack. In this case, the quality of the blood may be satisfactory, but it cannot get through to the heart-muscle cells, and thus cannot carry its benefits to them. The heart cells die and, as a result, all cells in the body finally die.

This is another example in which failure of cells to get what they need on one area can cause severe damage elsewhere in the body.

There are various special organs in the body that have special and distinctive nutritional requirements. All the hormone-producing glands in the body: the thyroid gland, the pituitary, the adrenals, the sex glands, the insulin-producing cells in the pancreas, the parathyroids, are made up of living cells which, like all other living cells, need continuous and complex nourishment. In addition, these cells need raw materials to build the respective hormones.

One of these hormones is particularly interesting because it contains a specific chemical element — iodine. The cells that produce the thyroid hormone are among the differentiated cells in the body: They absolutely need iodine if they are to perform their unique function. In certain parts of the world, such as the Great Lakes region, the Pacific Northwest, and Switzerland, iodine is at a low level in soil and vegetation. As a result, the thyroid glands of animals (dogs) and human beings are starved (relatively) for iodine; they become diseased, and highly swollen, thus calling attention to themselves (endemic goiter). They simply cannot do the job of producing the hormone adequately unless they are furnished enough iodine to put into it. When sufficient iodine is furnished through sea vegetation (kelp, Irish-moss, etc.) or the eating of fish from salt water, the enlarged thyroid gland reduces to normal size and the diseased condition disappears. By limiting the different degrees of the amount of iodine furnished a mammal, it is possible to produce severe simple goiter or any condition intermediate between this and completely normal functioning.

THE EFFECT OF FOOD ON THE MIND

At first glance, no connection between food and thinking is apparent; yet I assure you that, just as surely as food affects the different parts of the body, it also affects our thinking, for the very same reasons that pertain to the body. Our thought processes are influenced directly by what we have eaten; perhaps not from what we have last eaten, but surely from what we eat habitually.

The brain is given credit for the processes of thought, though some profess to doubt this, and maintain that thought originates outside of us, in the ethereal universe. But wherever it originates, the processes are certainly run by some parts of the body. The brain occupies the most strategic position in the body for direction of impulses; it is the logical seat for emotions, motivating impulses, and conscious thinking.

The brain is the great reflex center, from which radiate all the nerves that control motion and sensation; and as the brain must depend on the body for blood and oxygen, surely it must be affected by what we eat; for what we eat determines the sort of blood we have.

A brain nourished by blood laden with various toxic acid debris is surely not in a condition or position to function at its greatest efficiency. Toxic states can so befuddle the brain that clear thinking is impossible, and even deep comatose states will result from unusually deep types of intoxication, as we often observe.

To have a crystal-clear, alert, keen, sharp brain you must keep the toxic poisons of the blood at the lowest level and you must eat a diet that will supply every cell in the brain with the proper nourishment.

This calls for regular periods of fasting to keep the toxic poisons at the lowest levels and a diet that supplies all the nutrients required by the brain.

REFINED AND PROCESSED MODERN FOOD PRODUCES MANY BACKWARD CHILDREN

To show you the effect of toxic poison and malnutrition on the children of today, I have talked to many educators across the country, who have thousands upon thousands of children between the ages of six to seventeen that just cannot be educated. Their brains are sick from toxic poison and malnutrition because of our so-called standard American diet. These children have been fed on breakfast foods that have had all the nutrients refined out of them. Although the schools are blamed for turning out uneducated students, it is not the fault of the school teacher. The blame lies on the children's parents.

Mothers who buy and prepare food for the children are misled by T.V., radio, magazine and newspaper advertising. They tell the mothers to give the children canned soups which are composed of refined starch, sugar, and fat, that are rich in "empty calories" which quickly satisfies a child's appetite, but contain practically no minerals, vitamins, enzymes, roughage, or protein. They are told to give the children "Blunder bread" and "Ghost toasties" that have been "enriched". This is virtually an admission that essential food values have been extracted in the processing, and that the product needs to be "enriched". The mothers are told to put hot dogs, and lunch meats in this refined, bleached, bread. Both hot dogs and all lunch meats have two or more chemical additives. Children of today are allowed cola drinks and pop. They are filled with "empty calories" which may give a short surge of quick energy, but which have no basic nutrients such as vitamins and minerals. They eat commercial ice cream which is filled with all kinds of additives and commercial fillers, they eat candy bars, cookies, cakes, rich crackers, and pastries. These foods are called "deprived" foods. They satisfy a child by making him feel well-fed when he is truly being partly starved by spoiling his appetite for better, more nourishing foods.

How in heaven's name can you feed a child's brain on such "junk foods" as potato chips, and French fried potatoes with gobs of catsup smeared over them?

MOST AMERICAN YOUNG MEN UNFIT

Is it any wonder that 58 percent of all the young men who come up for military service are physically unfit?

Lt. Col. George Watson, USA, Planning Officer for Selective Service, stated on December 8, 1962: "Even though standards have not been raised, there is a worsening condition as it relates to American youth. The percentages of failures due to their inability to meet minimum draft requirements has been alarming".

The American Journal of Clinical Nutrition for April '61, flatly states that: "Nutrition is the most important single factor affecting health. This is true at age one or 101. But too often this fact is overlooked in the development of new health programs. Nutrition is a specific factor in the prevention and in the control of many chronic diseases".

Medical Science, May 25, '57 — "One out of every 14 boys and one out of every 17 girls under the age of 20 are hospitalized in a course of a year, according to the experience of one insurance company".

An editorial in the London Times said "The food industry, it predicts ... is in for a turbulent time and had better take steps at once to remedy its shameful neglect of basic research in nutrition''.

WORLD MEDICAL JOURNAL, Nov. '61. Dr. G. E. Burch, Prof. of Medicine, Tulane University, New Orleans, La., states ... ''Even in the young age-group, the incidence of neoplastic diseases such as leukemia is increasing. The collagen diseases such as acute arthritis are becoming more common.''

Boys made a sad showing in physical examinations; the nutritional status of girls — the mothers of tomorrow — is even more serious. Most nutritionists, doctors, and teachers agree that, basically, two factors are to blame; dietary ignorance and the lack of parental direction. One of the consequences is the inability to resist infectious disease. Childbirth complications are another result of poor nutrition. A girl whose nutrition is not adequate for her own body cannot expect to develop a health baby.

Americans consume more chemicals in their food than any other nation. At the same time, American forecasts are the gloomiest in the world about the continued rise of all the degenerative diseases.

The United States leads the civilized world in degenerative diseases, and in chemicalized foods. She also leads the world in high living standards and ample foods, which should reduce instead of increase the degenerative diseases.

THE SAD PHYSICAL AND MENTAL CONDITION
OF OUR ADULT POPULATION

If you think school-age children are befuddled in their thinking, let's look at the adult population. If you think the young population is half-sick or all-sick, our adult population is even worse.

I have stated that 58 percent of our youth from 18 to 25 are unfit for military service. If we examined our adult population from 25 to 75, what a group of physical and mental wrecks we would find.

If a group of fifteen adults are gathered together in a room for a social evening and the conversation turns to health and disease ... you can be sure that 99 percent of these people have some chronic ailment eating away at one or more vital organs. It seems that each one has something wrong with him. They talk of the shots they are taking, the operations they have had or are going to have ... the pills they are taking ... or the misery they are suffering. They calmly admit to each other that they are mentally disturbed, as if it were natural to be in that condition.

The longer the adult person lives on the standard civilized program the worse he gets, mentally and physically.

This proves out by the great number of convalescent nursing homes all over the country. These places are packed with prematurely-aging adults who are senile, feeble, forgetful, pitiful humans.

I ask you "Is this the way that God and Nature intended us to end our days on earth?"

If you are going to eat a diet deficient in the essential nutrients and you are going to let your body become loaded with vile, acid poisons, the answer is "yes."

Just because we live a limited number of years, there is absolutely no need that we break down, mentally and physically.

Since the mind is supported by purely physical processes, it is not hard to see the connection between foods and thinking; for the physical processes depend so completely on the character of foods eaten that it is not logical to disassociate the mind from foods.

During fasts, when the body nears a purified state, the mind is on such a high level that the subconscious mind becomes very active, and one can almost see through the occult. Some of the greatest mental feats have been performed during a fast, and a high degree of mental efficiency has been noted for rather long periods following the fast. Because fasting clears the system of much toxic debris, the brain is nourished with a much purer blood stream, and rises to amazing heights of efficiency.

We have achieved miracles in mechanics, invention, and science; but how much more might we have achieved if we had known the simple facts of proper nutrition as a background for thinking more efficiently.

The ancient philosophers of Greece placed proper diet first in training their students, and their rigid economy in the use of foods shows clearly the importance of this subject in their philosophy.

Epicurus, Socrates, Plato, and many others, placed great stress on food and its relation to the mind as a background for philosophic study; and they themselves practiced what they preached.

The philosophy of these sages is still respected today on a very high plane, even after the passing ages; and it has been said that some of the utterances of these men contain wisdom that seemed so far in advance of their times as to appear inspired.

Out of a foul body comes foul thoughts, and conversely, a clean, purified body emits clean thoughts; so much of the responsibility for clear thinking rests on the manner of feeding, however remote this connection may seem to those who have not seen the relationship demonstrated in many hundreds of cases of various types.

As the body becomes cleared of toxic acid debris, thinking is at once on a much higher plane; and the baser thinking, the grosser pleasures, seem to be idle and useless during this time.

"As a man thinketh in his heart, so is he," is more than a trite saying, and is capable of active and most convincing proof. When the body is cleared of this waste material, the mind soars to heights not formerly glimpsed by toxic minds, and new worlds seem to open to the fortunate one.

Most of the worthwhile things of life, those things that have elevated others, that have lived as great accomplishments for ages, have been achieved by those who placed accomplishment before idle pleasure! Among these benefactors, you will never find gluttons ... and will seldom ever find people who eat a devitalized, processed, or dead-food diet.

Eating is and should be a science, and one of the greatest importance to everyone, for it is such a fundamental thing. So much depends on it for efficiency, health, happiness, accomplishment, and the length of time we will remain on earth, that it should have much more important aspects in every person's early training.

It is never too late to start a program of wholesome nutrition. The very second you begin a natural diet ... your body, mind, and spirit starts to improve! In just eleven short months, you can build a whole, new, wonderful, youthful-feeling body, by fasting to clean out the half-dead cells and using natural foods to build new youthful cells. This is the great secret of life.

You will become the Master Builder of a brand new body ... free from miseries.

You will develop a sharp and alert brain.

Your spirit, your soul, the God-self within you will soar to greater heights.

There is no greater treasure than living on the highest planes of the physical, mental, and the spiritual.

Dr. Good Natural Food will be your guide to achieve the Higher Life. Trust him ... he wants you to have a perfect life while you are on earth.

Note: On page 173 you will find a complete guide to eating for the Higher Life. Study it carefully ... live by it and great benefits will be yours.

★ ★ ★ ★ ★

If you have health, you probably will be happy, and if you have health and happiness, you will have all the wealth you need, if not all you want.

- Elbert Hubbard

★ ★ ★ ★ ★

"Health is a state of mind in which the
body is not consciously present to use;
the state in which it is a joy to think,
to feel, to be, to see. "

- Sir Andrew Clark M. D.
Physician to Queen Victoria

★ ★ ★ ★ ★

Use your feet as Nature intended. Give them every possible freedom. Go barefoot every chance you get.

★ ★ ★ ★ ★

"They are as sick that surfeit with too much,
as they that starve with nothing. "

- Merchant of Venice, Shakespere

★ ★ ★ ★ ★

Why go globe-trotting for a healthful climate? Why not make your home a healthful place in which to live?

144

Fasting is accepted and recognized as being the oldest form of therapy. It is mentioned 74 times in the Bible. It is the universal therapy used by animals in the wilds the world over. As we study the ancient healers of the world, we find that fasting heads the list for helping Nature heal the sick and the wounded. There has been a misconception about fasting that must be clarified. It must be definitely and positively stated that fasting is not a cure of any disease or ailment. The purpose of the fast is to allow the body full range and scope to fulfill its self-healing, self-repairing, self-rejuvenating functions to the best advantage. Healing is an internal biological function. Fasting gives the body a physiological rest and permits the body to become 100 percent efficient in healing itself. Fasting under proper care or with workable knowledge is probably the fastest and the safest way or means of regaining health ever conceived by the human man.

If I have to repeat myself, I want to make it clear and positive that fasting does not cure anything. Fasting puts the body in a condition where all the Vital Force of the body is used to flush out the causes of body miseries. Fasting helps the body help itself. We who have made a life study of The Science of Fasting and conducted and supervised thousands of fasts, know the miracle that the body itself can perform during the period of complete abstinence from food. It gives the over-worked, over-burdened internal organs rest and time for rehabilitation. It exhilarates the internal power and vitality of the body to flush out toxic poisons and wastes that have been stored in the body for years. It raised the Vital Power to the highest point of efficiency. Thus it promotes the elimination of inorganic chemical accumulations and other pollutions that cannot be flushed from the body by any other means.

The prophets of old fasted for spiritual illumination and a closer contact with the Godhead (Divine Force). We know that fasting sharpens and makes the mental facilities keen and sharp. Fasting improves the organs of mastication, digestion, assimilation and elimination of food. The liver, which is known as the chemical laboratory of the human body and the most abused organ, has a chance during the fast to rehibilitate and pick up more Vital energy. Thus, after a fast the liver functions more efficiently. Particularly all the sensory powers possessed by human beings are exhilarated and raised to a much higher efficiency level than normal during and after a fast. No process of therapy ever fulfilled so many indications for restoration of vigorous health as does fasting. It is Nature's very own prime process, her first requirement in nearly all cases. After a fast the circulation is better, food can be assimilated better, vital vigor is greater, endurance, stamina and strength. After a fast the mind becomes more receptive to logic and a sensible natural way of living.

After the fast the mind becomes so powerful that it can take full control of the body. It becomes the complete master and if a person does not go back to his old habits, he can carry this mastery of the body for the rest of his life. Fasting gives a person confidence. Fasting gives a person a positive mental attitude. Fasting brings tranquillity of mind and a glow of well-being that no other therapy can achieve.

Fasting renovates, revivifies, and purifies each and every one of the millions of cells that make up the human body.

Fasting is the Royal Road to Internal Purity.

★ ★ ★ ★ ★

Fasting has been prominent as a means for intensifying prayer. Those who have found spiritual value during times set aside for prayer and fasting are found both in Scripture and throughout church history. Those who knew the values and secrets of fasting as a vital dimension in God included: Jesus Himself, the Apostle Paul, the early church leaders, Daniel, Elijah, Ezra, Esther, David, Hannah, Isaiah, Nehemiah, Zechariah and others. Prominent fasters in the annals of church history include John Calvin, Martin Luther, John Knox, John Wesley, David Brainard, George Muller, Rees Howells, and many more.

They discovered that abstaining from food not only freed them to focus upon God with fresh intensity, but opened avenues of spiritual perception and understanding that were not available during the rush of routine living. They found as they focused upon God by deliberate discipline, God focused upon them in clarity of direction and quickening of spirit. They could partake of God more easily with all else set aside.

Thy words were found, and I did eat them; and thy word was unto me the joy and rejoicing of mine heart: for I am called by thy name, O Lord God of hosts.

--Jeremiah 15:16

So we fasted and besought our God for this, and he listened to our entreaty.

--Ezra 8:23

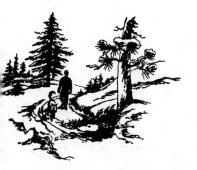

26

DOCTOR EXERCISE

Dr. Exercise makes these statements, "To rest is to rust" and rust means decay and destruction. In other words, the good doctor tells us that activity is LIFE, stagnation is death. The good doctor further tells us, that if we do not use our muscles, we lose them! In order to keep muscles firm, strong, vigorous, and youthful, they must be continually used. Activity is the Law of Life! Action is the Law of Well-Being. Every vital organ of the body has its specialized work, upon the performance of which its development and strength depend.

When we use the body, we build endurance, strength, and vigor. When we become lazy and do not use our muscles, we bring on decay and death. Daily exercise quickens and equalizes the circulation of the blood, but in laziness, the blood does not circulate freely and the changes in it that are so vital to life and health do not take place, and we have poor muscle tone. The muscles become flabby, sick, and unable to take vigorous activity.

People who do not exercise regularly have poor skin tone. In exercise, we bring on healthy perspiration in the 96 million pores of our body. The skin is the largest eliminative organ in the entire body. If someone would shellac or gild your body and thus clog the pores, you would die within a few minutes. With exercise, you bring on healthy perspiration Impurities and toxic poisons are expelled when you are exercising and perspiring freely, and you are allowing the skin to perform its natural function of eliminating poisons, If you do not exercise

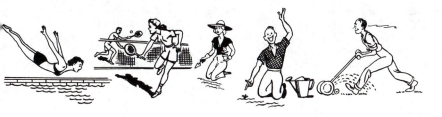

daily to the point of perspiration, all the work that the pores are not doing, throws a double burden on the other eliminative organs and then you get into trouble, physically. Vigorous exercise helps to normalize blood pressures; it helps to bring a healthy pulse. Vigorous exercise is an anticoagulant, which means that it keeps the blood from clotting (called a "thrombus") which often brings on a heart attack.

Every creature, human or otherwise, seeking to eliminate the internal waste, does so by means of muscular action. Inside your intestinal tract there are 3 muscular layers which undergo a rhythmic, wave-like action called peristalsis.

If you allow the internal and external muscles, through inactivity, to become flabby and fat instead of muscular, a serious condition results. The muscles lose their tonicity and power to contract, and the result is intestinal clogging. The abdominal muscles play an important role in the evacuation effort. What happens when the internal and external muscles become flabby, soft, sick and infiltrated with fat? They refuse to work, so we pile up intestinal waste that should have been eliminated. This brings about autointoxication, or the building of large amounts of toxic poison. I repeat that inactivity is the fruitful cause of many diseases.

Fasting, and diet are allies in your struggle for long-lasting youth, health, and symmetry. When it comes to fighting fat ... diet and fasting come first, but when it comes to keeping fit, it is exercise that matters most. However, they all help each other, for by taking exercise you may be more generous in your diet, and, up to a certain point, your food increase will make for increased vitality. The human machine should work at the highest pitch of efficiency. As with all machines, it improves with intelligent use, and nothing betrays its weak spots like inactivity and rust.

WALKING FOR LIFE

I believe in all of the many forms of exercise, but without hesitation, I will tell you that walking is the best all-around exercise.

Of all forms of exercise, walking is the one that brings most of the body into action. As you walk, grasp yourself in the small of the back, and feel how the entire frame responds to every stride, and how almost all of your chief muscles are functioning rhythmically. In no other exercise do we get the same harmony of coordinating sinews, and the same perfect circulation of blood. Walking is the king of exercise, and ideal for you.

Your walking should never be done consciously. No heel and
toe business. No getting there in a certain time. Let it be,
as it is, the most functional of exercises. Of course, you will
carry yourself well. Walk naturally with the head high, back
hollow, chest out, and because you will feel physically elated,
you will carry yourself proudly, straight, erect and with an
easy arm-swing.

Vow to become a wonderful walker, and make the day's walk a
fixed item in your health program all the year round, and in
any kind of weather. Go at your own stride with your spirit
free. If the outer world of nature fails to interest you, turn to
the inner world of the mind. For, as you walk, your body
ceases to matter and you become as near poet and philosopher
as you will ever be. Each to his taste, but to my mind this is
better than golf. Life has so much to teach us that it is a pity
to waste big chunks of time trying to get a ball into a hole in a
stroke less than the other fellow. However, the end is the
same — healthily-functioning muscles and quickened blood circulation with its attendant sense of harmony and happiness.

Gardening, too, is a marvelous form of exercise. It will give
you enough exercise in the open to keep you in the pink of physical condition. But you can get fat while gardening, because
there is too little movement, and you are bent over instead of
being erect. For this reason, I prefer walking. But perhaps
a little of both is best for you. Satisfy your conscience by
applying your energy productively in your garden, then take
the kink out of your back with a healthy walk.

In my personal life, I combine a system of calisthenics, plus
brisk walking and running.

IMPORTANCE OF ABDOMINAL EXERCISES

I believe the most important exercises are those that stimulate
all of the muscles of the human trunk from the hips to the arm-
pits. These are the binding muscles which hold all of the vital
organs in place, for, in developing your torsal muscles, you
are also developing the vital muscles. As your back, waist,
chest, and abdomen increase in soundness and elasticity, so
will your lungs, liver, heart, stomach, and kidneys gain in
efficiency.

The widened arch of your ribs will give free play to the lung
bellows, your elastic diaphragm will let the heart pump
and function more powerfully; your rubber-like waist will, in
its limber action, stimulate your kidneys and massage your liver.
Your abdominal muscles will strengthen and support your
stomach with controlled undulations. All of this hard, clean

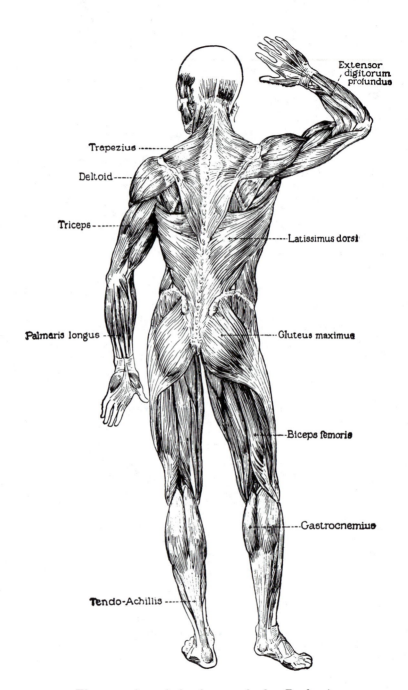

Extensor
digitorum
profundus

Trapezius

Deltoid

Triceps

Latissimus dorsi

Palmaris longus

Gluteus maximus

Biceps femoris

Gastrocnemius

Tendo-Achillis

The muscles of the human body. Back view.

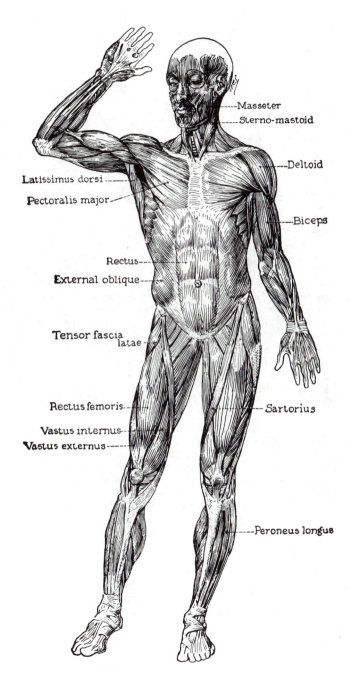

Masseter
Sterno-mastoid
Deltoid
Latissimus dorsi
Pectoralis major
Biceps
Rectus
External oblique
Tensor fascia latae
Rectus femoris
Sartorius
Vastus internus
Vastus externus
Peroneus longus

The muscles of the human body. Front view.

development of your torso will stimulate the sound walls of your house, which fortify the interior to resist the ravages of time. Trunk exercise is like a massage of the vital organs, and, for that reason, it has an influence over the whole organism that cannot be underestimated.

The more you fast, the more poison you will clean from your body and, as your body increases in internal cleanliness, so will your muscles have more tone and vitality.

You will find after a fast that the old logy, lazy feeling will leave you and, in its place, there will be a desire for more action, and more physical activity.

SHALL WE EXERCISE DURING FASTING ?

This is a question which only the faster can answer. If during a fast there is no inclination for physical activity, then you should not exercise. The fast is giving you a physiological rest and, unless there is a tremendous, overwhelming urge for physical activity, you should rest as much as possible. Your body is using all of its Vital Power for internal purification, but if you should feel, during a 7- to 10-day fast, that you need some stretching or walking, respond to the urge, by all means. It is between fasts and in your daily program of living that you should spend a portion of every day of your life, preferably in out-of-door exercises. Between the fasts, you may substitute vigorous circulation for a sluggish circulation. And a sluggish circulation is the cause of much discomfort, pain, and misery in the body.

When people do not exercise, their ankles and legs often swell because there is not enough blood circulating to remove the waste from the cells and carry it back to the organs of elimination. There should be no excuse for not exercising, because, regardless of your physical condition, it is most important that exercise be a part of your life. Daily exercise results in averting sickness and premature aging. It builds a fund of endurance and resistance. It helps to build a rich, red blood stream, giving you the proper balance of both white and red corpuscles to attack and overcome many harmful "bugs" that invade the body.

Exercise helps to maintain a serene and tranquil mind. A 5-mile walk in the fresh air will help to neutralize any unhealthful emotional upset. Exercise increases confidence for there is no better way to supreme confidence than the satisfying knowledge of an improved mental and physical ability. Exercise gives you a positive attitude. It cultivates the will and it gives absolute mastery of your Physical, Mental, and Spiritual Self and promotes personal efficiency. Exercise is the greatest health tonic one can take. You will attain this feeling of radiant, glorious living by fasting and exercise and you will feel better and look better. A body that craves physical activity must also produce the miraculous feeling of AGELESSNESS.

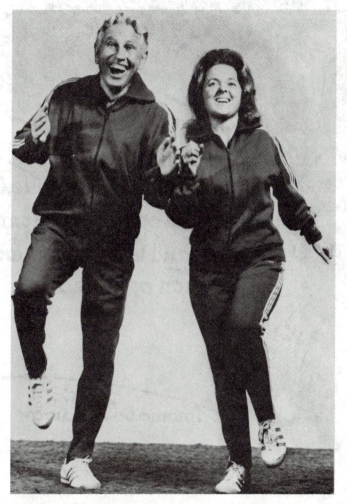

Paul Bragg and daughter Patricia at the start of their vigorous daily morning exercise program to keep in peak physical condition.

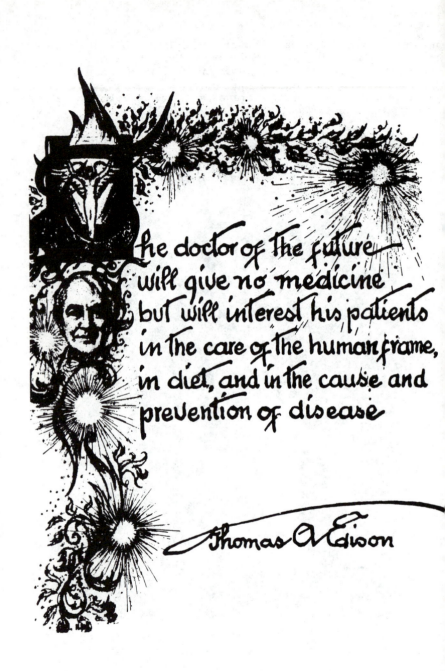

The doctor of the future
will give no medicine
but will interest his patients
in the care of the human frame,
in diet, and in the cause and
prevention of disease

Thomas A Edison

154

27

DOCTOR 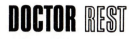REST

Dr. Rest is another specialist always at your command to help you win Vitality Supreme. I believe the word "rest" is the most misunderstood word in the dictionary. Some people's idea of resting is to sit down and drink a cup of strong stimulant, such as alcohol, coffee, tea, or soft drinks. This is so well portrayed in the modern coffee break for employees. To me, rest means repose, freedom from activity, quiet, tranquillity. It means peace of mind and spirit, it means to rest without anxiety or worry, and it means to refresh one's self. Your rest should be a general refresher of your whole nervous system.

It does not mean sitting with one leg crossed over the other, because when you sit in this position, you are putting a tremendous burden on the artery which supplies the feet with blood and also cuts off nerve energy. So if you sit with one leg crossed over the other, you are not resting, you are giving the heart a tremendous load of work to do. Don't cross your legs when you sit down — keep both feet on the floor!

To rest means to allow a free circulation of blood in the entire body. If your shoes are too tight, if your collar is too tight, if your hat is too tight, if your belt or any of your undergarments are too tight, if garters or stockings are too tight, you are not resting when you sit still or lie down.

The best rest is secured when all of the clothes are off the body. Any clothes, you are wearing should be comfortably loose and never binding.

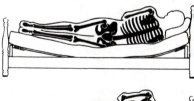

Bad Resting - Sagging Bed

Good Resting - Firm Bed

Why do we rest? You often hear people say "I must have a rest". But when they sit down to rest, they nervously thump their fingers on a table or desk, or they squirm or move restlessly. The art of resting is something that must be acquired and concentrated upon. Among the various ways you can rest is to lie down on a firm bed or couch unclothed or with as few loose clothes as possible. One of the finest ways to rest is a sun bath, because, if there is anything that will relax the muscles and nerves, it is the soothing rays of the sun. As you rest, you must learn to clear your mind of all anxiety, worries, and emotional problems. When the muscles and nerves are relaxed, the heart action slows, and especially when you take long, slow, deep breaths. This will bring deep relaxation and total rest.

Another form of resting is a short nap, and in taking this nap, you should command your muscles to become completely relaxed. Your conscious and subconscious mind control the muscles and the nerves, so you must be in complete command of your body when you rest. The Master Teacher, and His Disciples, when worn and weary, said "Come Ye and Rest a While." The Master did not lead them into the busy streets of Jerusalem where there was noise and clatter. He didn't even take them into the synagogue, but into the quiet of the wide open spaces, under the blue sky. Here He could rebuild, relax, and revivify every organ of their exhausted bodies, and revitalize, refresh, and invigorate their weary minds. Under the blue sky in the clean, fresh air is the greatest place to relax and rest, and renew your Vital Force.

To me, sleep is the greatest revitalizer we have, but so few people get a long, peaceful, and refreshing night's sleep. Most people habitually use stimulants; tobacco, drugs, coffee, tea, alcohol, and cola drinks. All of these whip the tired nerves, so that people who use these stimulants never have complete rest and relaxation, because their nerves are always in an excited condition. Most people do not earn their rest; rest is something that must be earned with physical and mental activity, because they go hand in hand. So many people have come to me, telling me what poor sleepers they were, and how they roll and toss all night long. Today, thousands of people are forced to take some type of drug to induce sleep, but this is not true sleep. No one can get restful sleep with a drug. You may drug yourself to unconsciousness, but you cannot drug yourself to a restful, normal, healthful, and satisfying sleep.

A body full of toxic poisons is a continual irritant to the nerves. How is it possible to get a good nights rest with irritated nerves? I have found in my years of experience with fasting, that when people discard their stimulants while on a fasting program, tl become deep, restful sleepers. You will notice as you purify your body that you will be able to relax more readily. You will be able to nap often, and you will enjoy the benefits of a long, restful, night's sleep. Rest is important! The Bible tells us that God appointed one day of rest every week for man. In this act of God Almighty, we have plenty of support for our contention that frequent change of activity is an important factor in the maintenance of super-health. Along with our busy days, we must add some form of recreation to our activities. We have all heard the trite saying "All work and no play makes Jack a dull boy."

Today we live in a mad, competitive world which in business parley is called "The Rat Race". In our civilization, it is dog-eat-dog, so we build up tremendous pressures, tensions, stresses, and strains. I believe this is the reason why people turn to tobacco, drugs, coffee, alcohol, and other stimulants. There is not only competition in the business world, but status must be upheld. People are always trying to impress one another, and trying to create an image. Thus a false image is created and it takes a tremendous amount of energy to portray a false image! There is competition among women, who have been told that gray hair makes them look old, so they spend hours having their hair colored, to constantly keep up with the latest fashions, which also calls for energy. Our whole modern civilization is one that "whip-drives" and pushes us.

LIFE IS TO BE ENJOYED!

It is no wonder that we have created fifteen million chronic alcoholics, and millions of drug addicts. Have we completely forgotten that life is to be lived, to be enjoyed? Leisure living is something few people in our modern society enjoy. Life is rush, rush, and more rushing; where are we rushing to? Where? To the hospital or the graveyard?

To be able to relax, rest, and sleep, your day must be programmed to have time for rest, recreation, exercise, and a good night's sleep. You cannot get a good night's sleep if you overload your stomach. You cannot have a good night's sleep unless you have had some vigorous out-of-door exercise such as a 2-mile brisk walk or garden work. I do not consider housework or the daily occupation as the way to get exercise and activity. Let your body be nourished by pure, natural food and distilled water ... let it have plenty of fresh air and sunlight. Have a balanced program of exercise and repose and let Nature do the rest; treat yourself as if you were a fine beast of pure-bred stock, and as surely as it will win prizes for superiority, so will you! It is all too easy to sneer and laugh at the "back to Nature" people, but we who believe in Nature will always have the last laugh.

GET THE SENSE OF NATURE

One of the predominant suggestions of this book, then, is a gradual return to a more natural way of living. In food, clothing, rest, sleep, and a simplicity in living habits, try to reach a nearness to Nature that makes you almost one with her.

When you feel that the same pure forces that express themselves in a pine tree are expressing themselves in you, you have made a big stride toward a health ideal.

Begin to live as Nature wants you to live. Seek to feel that she claims you and that you are part of glad, growing things. Put yourself into her hands and let her have her way with you. Leave to the young the smog-filled, air-polluted, microbe-infested cities. You will find that in the quiet beauty of hill and meadow, you will rekindle your own youth. If you would grow young, begin by believing you can, and that Nature is eager to aid you. Better than any human or divine agency, she can run that ill-used machine of yours, and, if it breaks down while in her hands, it is because its usefulness is really at an end.

If you are a prisoner of a city, make it a point to get out in the country or the sea shore where you can really find true rest, tranquillity, and serenity.

In a brotherly way, I have tried to stress these points. First, you should demand of yourself a higher standard of health and happiness. You cannot receive higher health unless your body gets its rest periods to develop new vitality and energy. Second, you should regard your body as a machine under your care and control, and every machine must have rest periods. If not, you will build up too much friction — that is what we do in our lives — we build up too much nerve irritation. Third, with increasing years, you should draw closer and more intimately to Nature. You should cease to look for thrills and over-stimulation, and instead, seek a life of serenity and peacefulness. By living in simplicity and purity, you will be as healthy as a carrot in the Bragg organically-grown garden.

Let health, air, sun, and complete rest work for you. With a serene clear eye, and confidence, put yourself in Nature's hands. Let her run your machine, heal your hurts, comfort you in sickness and adversity. Then, when you have lived a long life of usefulness and happiness, let her call you back home. Make Nature your partner, and when you are resting, relaxing, and recreating new energy, Nature will always be there with her kind hand on your shoulder. So be a child of Nature, don't look for sophisticated thrills, but find your fun and diversion in relaxation and other pursuits that are simple, down to earth, and one with Nature. Your rewards will be many, in renewed health, a calmness of spirit, and a new awareness of the perfect natural beauties that Nature has bestowed upon us so generously.

RELAX — IT'S NO CRIME

In our American Culture, we are prone to look down on the person who wants to relax, or live a leisurely life. It seems that we must be doing something constantly. We must be reading, talking, listening to music, or watching television. We have to attend dances, parties, movies, programs, and athletic sports. We are constantly pushing and driving our bodies. No wonder so many people have emotional problems, and no wonder the psychiatrists and the psychologists are overworked. It is because we ourselves are overworked.

Please do not be ashamed to sit down or lie down and rest, or relax to get off the treadmill. It is not only fun to just do nothing, it is healthful and necessary.

You have a natural, built-in, tranquilizer system located throughout your body in the muscle cells, which you should be using. Don't expect to take sedatives and yet become skilled in relaxation. Barbiturates and true relaxation are not bedfellows. On the other hand, I have known persons who have needed sedatives for six months or longer and were able to discard them after going on a fasting program.

To relax yourself to sleep, first darken the room to some extent, turn off the T. V. or radio, and lie flat on your back with your hands down at either side without touching your body, to reduce sensory stimulation to a minimum. Let your hands rest, palms down, on the bed. Legs should be extended with the feet approximately a foot apart. Your head may rest on a small pillow or directly on the bed, whichever is more comfortable. Permit your eyes to remain open at first, looking at an area, not at a point directly in front of you, that is, on the opposite wall or ceiling, not up or down, or to either side. After the movements of your eyes have ceased, blinking movements of the lids may continue for a while. These will not interfere with the relaxation of the eye muscles.

Thinking is always accompanied by eye movements. By relaxing your eyelids and eye muscles, you are slowing down your thought processes — and the end result of relaxation of the eyes and of other parts of the body is a natural, quiet, and restorative sleep.

If you have insomnia, reading just before going to sleep, or reading to put yourself to sleep, is not helpful, because, in all likelihood, your eye muscles are already over-fatigued. Reading will tire them more, increasing the eye muscle tension, and interfering with the process of relaxation, which if uninterrupted would inevitably lead to sleep.

AVOID INTERRUPTIONS

Disregard all minor muscular discomfort while lying perfectly still, and permit all of your muscles (you have 840 voluntary muscles) to relax without interruption. Do not tighten or move any muscles unless absolutely necessary. Movements of an arm or leg, or a change in your position, will interrupt the entire relaxation process, and those muscles which have already attained a certain degree of relaxation must begin the process all over again. Muscles that are overly tense may be uncomfortable, but if you move them you will only prolong their discomfort. Permit them to relax and, in most instances, the distress will disappear within ten to fifteen minutes. A relaxed muscle is a comfortable muscle and if you are relaxing efficiently, you will feel comfortable. Discomfort in a muscle or muscle group is an indication that it is tense, that you are not permitting it to relax.

FALSE NOTIONS

In the practice of relaxation, beginners have told me many times that they cannot possibly lie on their backs and go to sleep in that position. In observing the training of several hundred individuals, I have yet to prove the truth of that statement. If this is your belief, disregard it, for no matter how deeply entrenched this idea may be in your mind, you will be able to prove it is fallacious.

"I always have to sleep on my right side." "I always sleep on my stomach." "I must curl up when I sleep." "I have to change my position frequently." "I cannot sleep at night if I have a nap in the daytime." "I must have my hand resting on my stomach." "I can go to sleep when I go to bed, but I wake up around 2 or 3 A.M. and can't go back to sleep." "I sleep right through until 5 A.M., but then I am wide awake until I get up at 7 o'clock — and then I am tired out by afternoon." These are common complaints — but I have yet to find a person willing to devote 15 minutes a day in training himself to relax who cannot learn to break these habits, if they live by the natural system of living and a fasting program.

Insomnia usually responds to relaxation techniques within 10 days to two weeks, and then sweet, beautiful sleep will be yours every night and you will wake up in the morning as bright and fresh as a healthy newborn baby.

Your fasting program is going to help you secure complete rest, relaxation, and sound, sweet sleep. Toxins put pressure on nerves and muscles. Fasting releases these pressures and allows them to relax.

★ ★ ★ ★ ★

CREATIVE MEDICINE

It is no oversimplification to say that our health comes from the soil. No matter how many physicians and health officers we train, and how much curative or preventive medicine they may practice, we cannot attain optimum health until they and we have turned our attention to creative medicine, and thereby learn to keep and even improve our health. To build and maintain good soil is the real fundamental service. Creative medicine must be founded on growing the best foods. Thus alone can we create real health for our people--only through creating a sound and prosperous agriculture.

-Dr. Jonathan Foreman in "The Land."

★ ★ ★ ★ ★

MONDAY TO JOY-DAY

There are days when you feel buried in the blues. You get up feeling depressed and pessimistic. You look worried. The world just isn't spinning in your direction. Yesterday you had it on a string, but today it has you beneath its weight.

What to do? We should realize that we are destined to have these days. They are as natural as rain. If we were always happy we'd not appreciate our joys. If we didn't have hard knocks, we wouldn't appreciate the pleasant times so much. Maybe it takes Monday morning blues to make a week well-balanced.

-Dr. P. DeWitt Fox in "Health Culture"

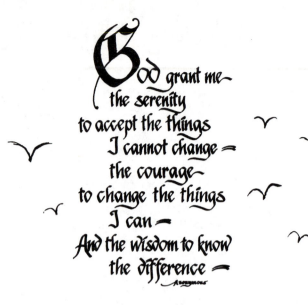

God grant me
the serenity
to accept the things
I cannot change —
the courage
to change the things
I can —
And the wisdom to know
the difference —

— Anonymous

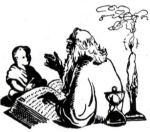

"Why not look for the best — the best in others, the best in ourselves, the best in all life situations? He who looks for the best knows the worst is there but refuses to be discouraged by it. Though temporarily defeated, dismayed, he smiles and tries again. If you look for the best, life will become pleasant for you and everyone around you."

— Paul S. Osumi

28

DOCTOR GOOD POSTURE

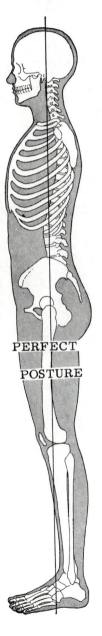

PERFECT

POSTURE

Why should emphasis be placed upon such a simple thing as the pull of gravity? This is very easy to explain. In the past, as long as your muscles were strong enough, they held your skeleton in proper balance with its many points and sections free from strain or dis-comfort. Now, however, your muscles are losing the battle with gravity. Maybe you are prematurely older, or heavier, or an enforced rest has weakened your muscles just enough to its present uncomfortable state of balance.

Such a sagging stretches the ligaments of your back and causes backache. Ligaments that are unduly stretched are painful. Ligaments are meant to serve only as check reins for the joints and they cannot be forcibly stretched without pain. When the ligaments in your back are made uncomfortable by stretching, it is only natural for your muscles to try to oppose the sagging of your back which results from the pull of gravity. However, your muscles are too weak to do their proper job, so they rapidly become exhausted and develop the rankling misery of fatigue, making your back even more uncomfortable. Check your own symptoms! Do you notice a deep aching and soreness along your spine due to stretched ligaments? Are your back and shoulder muscles achy and tired? Is yours a postural backache due basically to weak muscles? If it is, it's about time you did something sensible to relieve it — like strengthening those weak muscles by proper exercise.

Look at yourself in the mirror! Do your shoulders slump? Is your upper back round? Have you a potbelly? Are you a sway-back? Can you see the reasons, now, why your back has the right to ache? The bending, slump-ing, ligament-stretching force of gravity has finally taken charge. But even though you are presently a hapless sufferer of backache due to poor muscles and bad posture, do not

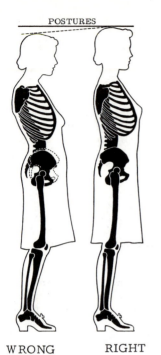

WRONG   RIGHT

despair. You can regain back comfort if weak muscles and poor posture are at fault!

It has been said that backache is the penalty man must pay for the privilege of standing and walking upright on two feet. Although man's ancestors are believed by some to have been four-footed creatures, there is no doubt about the fact that man himself is definitely two-footed. Every infant struggles instinctively to stand on his own two feet and walk. He need not be taught. He will attempt this biped gait even if left alone most of the time and never instructed. It is natural for a human being to stand and walk in this manner. This is interesting, because there are no animals which spend all of their standing and walking hours on two feet — not even the chimpanzees or the gorillas. These higher apes use their hands and arms to help them move about. The world's strongest gorilla would be unable to follow a fragile housewife about, walking as erectly as she does, for more than a short time. This is because human beings are meant to walk erect, and other animals are not.

The spines of human beings have normal curves which enable the muscles to oppose gravity and hold their backs erect. As long as the muscles are strong enough to maintain the balance of these curves and prevent sagging, the back is comfortable. When the muscles are too weak to do their normal work, the back sags, ligaments are stretched, and backache enters the picture.

To maintain one's self in a healthy state involves many factors; right natural food, rest, exercise, sleep, fasting, control of emotions and mind, and last but not least, good posture. If a body is well-nourished and cared for, good posture is not a problem. When the body lacks any of the essentials, poor posture is often the result. Once poor habits have been established, one must resort to definite and corrective measures, such as proper exercises and deliberate postural habits.

HOW TO STAND, SIT AND WALK FOR
STRENGTH AND HEALTH

When in a sitting position, see that the spine is well back against the chair and, again, that the abdominal cavity is not relaxed, but well drawn in, shoulders back, head high and never forward. The position can be with arms folded or the hands clasped in the lap.

When walking, one should imagine that the legs are attached to the middle of the chest and that gives long, sweeping, graceful, springy steps, because when one walks correctly with this swing and spring, he automatically builds energy. Habit either makes or breaks us, and good posture habits make graceful, strong bodies. "Just as the twig is bent, the tree is inclined."

When in a sitting position, never cross one leg over the other. Under the knees run two of the largest arteries, carrying nourishing blood to the muscles below the knee and to the thousands of nerves that are found in the feet. When you cross your legs, you immediately cut down the blood to almost a trickle. Therefore, when the muscles of the leg and knee are not nourished and do not have a good circulation, we go stagnant in the extremities which can lead to varicose veins, or broken capillaries. Look at the bare ankles of people 40 and over who have made it a habit of crossing their legs and see all the broken veins and broken capillaries. When the muscles and feet do not get their full supply of blood the feet become weak poor circulation sets in. Cold feet torment the leg-crosser.

A well known heart specialist was asked once, "When do most people have a heart attack?" The heart specialist answered, "At a time they are sitting quietly with one leg crossed over the other." So you can see that when you sit down you should plant both of your feet squarely on the floor and never cross

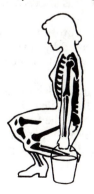

RIGHT LIFTING

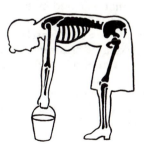

WRONG LIFTING

your legs. People who are habitual leg-crossers always have more acid crystals stored in the feet than those who never cross their legs while sitting. Crossing the legs is one of the worst postural habits of man. It throws the hips off balance, throws the spine off balance and throws the head off balance and can become one of the most prolific causes of a chronic backache. Poor posture of any kind can bring an unbearable pain across your upper back, fatigue in your drooping shoulders ... as well as soreness shooting from the base of your neck to the back of your throbbing head and downward to mingle with stiffness in the belt area of your lower back. Poor posture causes weakness in your hips and loins, a numb feeling at your tail bone, and a shooting pain down your legs. Bad posture can develop aches and pains not only in the back, but all over the body.

One very simple habit, but most beneficial one to establish, is to stand tall, walk tall, sit tall, never crossing one leg over the other. This does not require an exaggerated position, and when one stands tall, walks tall and sits tall, a correct posture is assumed and all of the sagging, dropped and pro-lapsed vital organs will assume normal position and function; that is, if all other natural habits of living are practiced every day.

★ ★ ★ ★ ★

Dr. Nikolayev, the director of the fasting unit - Moscow Psychiatric Institute - fasts several times a year in 10 to 15 day stret-ches. "I usually fast for prophylactic reasons," he stated. "I have fasted several times with a scientific purpose in view, to make an ex-periment. I always feel excellent when I fast. It is always a happy oc-casion and a rest for me."

Dr. Nikolayev often quotes an old German proverb: "The illness that cannot be cured by fasting cannot be cured by anything else." Fasting permits the considerable healing powers of the body and of the mind to assert themselves.

Dr. Nikolayev discovered that his patients responded to the Fasting treatment after all other forms of therapy had failed. The patients had been chronically ill and felt hopeless about the future. Most of them would never have functioned again. Seventy percent of those treated by fasting improved so remarkably that they were able to resume an active life.*

---

* FASTING the Ultimate Diet - Bantam Books, NY - Allan Cott M.D.

29

DOCTOR HUMAN MIND

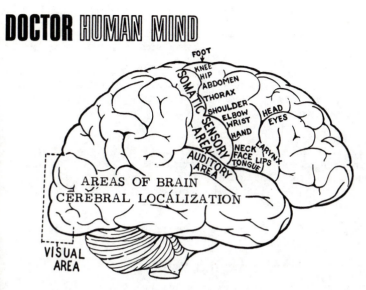

AREAS OF BRAIN
CEREBRAL LOCÁLIZATION

VISUAL AREA

MAN A TRINITY

There is an old German saying: "Alle gute Dinge sind Drei." or "All good things are three".

We worship a God represented by a trinity, the Father, Son, and Holy Ghost.

The soul is the head man, the first man, the ego, the individual, the personality, which makes each of us individuals.

The mind is the second man, through which the soul or the first man expresses; the soul's only means of expression.

The body is the third man, the physical, visible part; the means by which the mind expresses, also its only means, and its only mode of contact with environment.

These three are one, just as the Godhead (Divine Force) is one, each making up a part of this individual called man.

"The body is composed of many members, yet is one body."

"If one of the members suffer, all others suffer with it."

We recognize the body as an indivisible unit, a community of closely grouped and interrelated organs, tissues, and cells, each individual, yet so closely related that not one of them can exist apart from the whole.

The public has too long viewed these various organs as unrelated, or loosely related, units, and has been inclined to treat each more or less individually, not realizing that if one indivisible unit suffers, all the rest suffer with it.

The body is the most wonderful example of widely diversified functions in one indivisible whole that was ever conceived, and it must be treated always as a unit. What is good for one part is good for all; what is bad for one part is bad for all.

If the toe is affected by gangrene, does not the whole body suffer with it? Not only is the pain reflected to the whole man, but the absorption of decaying material has to be taken care of by the whole man; the loss of appetite, the headache, the nausea, the fever, and the chills; yet the toe is the only affected member that can be seen.

In the science of fasting, we are concerned with the whole man ... the soul, mind and body.

RIGHT THINKING AND HEALTH

In the book of Proverbs, the ancient Wise Man tell us, "For as he thinketh in his heart, so is he." (Proverbs 23:7)

When a sick person constantly convinces himself that he will never get well ... it becomes almost certain that he will carry his troubles to the grave.

FLESH IS DUMB. I never want you to forget that statement. That is the reason I use it over and over again. Your mind is really the controlling factor in your entire makeup.

Flesh cannot think for itself because only the mind does all the thinking. That is why you must cultivate only Positive thinking.

Your mind must rule your body with a will of iron. The mind must always be in command of the body.

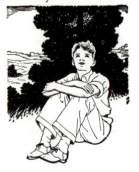

From this day on you must learn thought substitution ... when a negative thought such as "I am losing my sight because when you get older you start to lose sight" enters your mind ... substitute it for a positive thought that says "Age cannot in any way affect my sight. Age is not toxic."

Keep in mind always that what the mind tells dumb flesh, that is exactly what the flesh is going to believe and act upon. Mind influences flesh.

Let your mind make all the decisions for your body, because if your body rules your mind, you face a life of misery and slavery.

The "dope fiend" is the extreme example of the body ruling the mind. The body's craving for dope can force the mind to command the body to commit any crime of violence so that it may satisfy the body with the dope that it craves.

The same applies to alcohol, tea, coffee, and any other stimulant. The body does the ruling and not the mind.

We maintain most of our bad habits simply because our minds are enslaved by our bodies.

The body rules by the false philosophy of "Eat, drink and be merry, for tomorrow you die."

This is false. You don't die tomorrow, but you continue to live by this philosophy, and five, ten or twenty years later you are burdened into a sick, weak, premature-aging body that tortures you day and night.

Remember always, you are punished by your bad habits of living. Not for them, but by them. That is the law.

Sickness, aches, pains, and physical suffering are ills that YOU are responsible for personally. YOU committed the crimes against your body because you did not use your God-given reason and intelligence to rule your body with your mind, by living by the natural laws.

What has your psychology to do with Health and long life? Far more than the majority of men and women realize. Think of your thoughts as powers, as magnets, as entities which have the ability to attract or repel, according to the way they are used.

A great majority of people lean either to the positive or the negative side mentally; the former phase is constructive and tends in the direction of achievement, while the negative side of life is destructive, leading to futility and failure. It is self-evident that it is to everyone's advantage to cultivate a positive mental attitude. With patience and persistence this can be accomplished.

There are many negative or destructive forms of thought which react in every cell in your body. The strongest is fear, and its child, worry, along with depression, anxiety, apprehension, jealousy, envy, ill-will, covetousness, anger, rancor, resentment, revengefulness, and self-pity. All of these bring tension to the body and mind leading to waste of energy, enervation, and either slow or rapid poisoning of the body; rage, intense fear, and shock are very violent and quickly intoxicate the system; worry and other destructive emotions act more slowly, but, in the end, have the same effect. Anger and intense fear stop digestive action, upsetting also the kidneys and the colon. These are scientifically-demonstrated, physiological truths.

Fear and worry, as well as the other destructive phases of thought, muddle the mind. A crystal-clear mind is needed to reason to the best advantage, thus enabling us to make sound decisions. A beclouded mind must necessarily make inferior decisions, assuming it is able to reach any conclusions at all.

A HEALTHY MIND IN A HEALTHY BODY

What are the positive mental forces or expressions? They are the ones that lead to peace of mind, to inner relaxation, as opposed to the destructive ones which cause tightening-up of the entire system.

This very second, let your mind take over your body.

In your mind, form an image of the person you want to be. Now, with nature's nine doctors as your helpers, you can make yourself exactly what YOU want to be. Believe in the power of positive thinking. Practice thought-substitution ... never ever let a negative thought take over your mind. In this way, you set your own pattern of living, and you make your mind a powerhouse of constructive thoughts. Strengthen your mind so thoroughly that if any of your weak, fearful, relatives or friends tell you that fasting is starvation, and that something harmful can come out of your health program ... let your remarks slide out of your mind like water off a duck's back. Feel sorry for these poor, weak, fearful, ignorant people because you will live to see them perish and go to their graves long before their time.

- Each time you fast, you will make your mind stronger, and more positive.

- Each time you fast, you will eliminate fear and worry.

- Fasting helps you to a higher life. That is why the greatest spiritual leaders were ardent fasters.

170

- Fasting elevates the soul, the mind, and body. What greater rewards can you desire in life?

By fasting, you can create the person you have always longed to be. That is, if you demand only the best life can offer.

Only when the body and mind are in harmony will there be opportunity for proper spiritual development; never forget that the spiritual man is first, the mental, second, and the physical, the third man; and the only when the second and third are in harmony, can there be a proper spiritual life!

Spirituality depends far more on proper harmony of the rest of the man than is generally thought; and we all have it in our power to create this harmony through proper understanding of the relationship of these three entities, and the means necessary to keep them in harmony.

Use your mind to help you attain your desires by developing a constructive philosophy of life.

Think constructively about health, know what the requirements of wholesome living are, employ your mind and will power to live accordingly, and your determination to continue in that way, and health in soul, mind, and body will be yours.

Join hands with nature in making yourself a true living Trinity.

Fasting and a constructive program of Healthful Living can take you to the heights of true living that very few experience on this earth.

Let your mind take control of your body this instant. New doors will open for you. You will be leaving the darkness and living in the light. Darkness is death, light is life, so let in the brightness of the light of a good life, today!

★ ★ ★ ★ ★

"The greatest tragedy that comes to man is the emotional depression, the dulling of the intellect and the loss of initiative that comes from nutritive failure."
- Dr. James S. McLester
Former President A. M. A.

★★★★★★★★

"Men do not die, they kill themselves."
—Seneca, Roman Philosopher

For the kingdom of God is not meat and drink; but righteousness, and peace, and joy in the Holy Ghost.

--Romans 14:17

When thou fastest appear not unto men to fast, but unto thy Father which is in secret: and thy Father, which seeth in secret, shall award thee openly.

--Matthew 6:17, 18

Moreover, when ye fast.

--Matthew 6:16

Jesus lived by His own rules — He fasted.

And Jesus being full of the Holy Ghost returned from Jordan, and was led by the Spirit into the wilderness, being forty days tempted of the devil. And in those days he did eat nothing: and when they were ended, he afterward hungered.

--Luke 4:1,2

Fasting and prayer seemed to strengthen Jesus, for when His time of temptation and fasting was ended, He manifested a new adequacy and poise.

And Jesus returned in the power of the Spirit into Galilee . . .
--Luke 4:14

The ministry of Jesus among the people then began in earnest. Fasting had accomplished something.

That fasting is a normal part of our walk with God is taken for granted by the Lord Jesus. Immediately following the Lord's Prayer, He said: *Moreover when ye fast—*

--Matthew 6:16

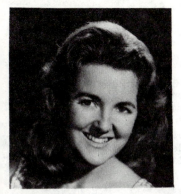

30

THE SCIENCE OF EATING FOR SUPERIOR HEALTH

It is the consensus of opinion among the average people that we must eat — "To keep up our strength". This association of food and strength has been so inculcated into man's subconscious mind that he feels he must eat three times a day of foods, "That stick to the ribs". We look upon a person who has a big appetite as a healthy person. If we know of a person who has been sick, we are always encouraged when he is able to sit up and take nourishment.

During my long research and study on the value of food, I have come to regard nourishment as something more than habitual eating. The body can be fed with anything that is put into the stomach to subdue hunger. Food, however, plays an important role in our lives because the body is built from the food we eat. With food we either build strong, disease-free, youthful cells or we build half-sick cells. Cells that do not support us as they should. So we must always eat food that builds sturdy, strong cells which are converted into body tissue. We see a lot of people who are well-fed, but they are far from well-nourished. The skin tone, the muscle tone, and the energy is not in these people, even though plenty of food is coming into their bodies.

At one time in man's history when his food came exclusively from the hands of Nature, unprocessed and undefiled by greedy man, man had a natural attraction to the kind of food his body needed, and had a superior sensitivity in his selection of food for life. In other words, there was an inner-voice that told him what to eat. We can call it instinct, or we can call it by any other name, but at one time in the early history of man, he was a beautiful specimen.

I believe that man originated in the tropics, his natural home, where his entire body was nourished by the powerful rays of the sun. We know that the skin needs Vitamin D, which is found in sunshine. We also know that the skin needs Vitamin A, but today man's body has become so degenerated, so filled with mucus, acid toxins and mineral and vitamin deficiencies that he can no longer live in the sunshine. There are many people who develop all kinds of skin conditions by exposure to the sun, and erroneously put the blame on the sunshine.

Man has degenerated his skin by the over-use of soap. I haven't used soap on my body for years, with the exception of lather on my face to shave, and to wash my hands when water fails to remove the accumulated dirt. So by man putting on clothes and going into the cold climates, he lost contact with the food supplied by the sun on his nude body. Civilized man smothers his body with heavy clothes.

I believe that in man's original home, the tropical paradise, his diet was made up of an abundance of raw fruits and vegetables, plus an abundance of all varieties of nuts and seeds. I believe it was on this diet that man was able to live for 900 years. His digestive system was perfectly attuned to his natural diet. Man, in his essential structure, has no weapons for killing, and I believe that the first people who inhabited the tropics of this earth were vegetarians.

However, I do not believe that it is possible for everyone to be a vegetarian today. Man of 5 or 6 thousand years ago was an entirely different creature than man today. In those days man went to the field and the forest where there was an abundance of life-giving food. Today man lives as a civilized being. We live in houses. We shut our bodies away from fresh air, and breathe in pollution. We drink chemically-treated water and do not get the physical exercise that early man enjoyed. Man in America today has only a life expectancy of 68 years, whereas, men before the great flood, lived for as long as 900 years.

We have lost our tropical paradise, and man today must live in his poisoned cities, drink his poisoned-water, breath polluted air and eat food that is picked half-ripe. In other words, the situation of original man and civilized man is far apart.

But we must do more than bemoan our lost Garden of Eden. We must face reality in all its ugliness.

FOR HEALTH — KEEP ON THE ALKALINE DIET

I want you to understand this as I present this program of eating to you. It is a program designed to give you the best nourishment that the food of civilization can offer you. At the same time, the suggested menus are also purification menus, that is, you must look upon all fruits and vegetables, not only as protective foods, not only as foods that are filled with minerals, vitamins, enzymes and valuable nutrients, but foods that are highly alkaline to help you keep down acidity.

Many people studying nutrition become confused because there are so many varying opinions. Some nutritionists advise a high protein diet, some nutritionists advise a low carbohydrate diet; there are nutritionists who advise a raw fruit diet; a vegetarian diet; a lacto-vegetarian diet. Each authority says that his is the best. I respect every scientist's views in the field of nutrition. He has come to these conclusions by study, research and observation. I believe that it is impossible to lay down absolute nutritional laws except when it comes to eliminating the dead, devitalized, demineralized, processed, sprayed and calorie-empty foods of our present day civilization.

Today we have a selection of approximately 200 foods. Around these 200 foods you can build an adequate diet. As you fast you will purify your body and as you purify your body, your body itself will make a selection of foods. The main thing is to eliminate the perverted foods of modern civilization. It is not so much what you eat as what you shouldn't eat. On page 186 of this book I have given you the list of foods to avoid. There is an old trite saying "A man is either his own doctor at 40 or he is a fool". May I say here that I believe that any person 30 years of age who is not his own dietitian is going to run into some very serious physical trouble.

Our physical and mental activity draws heavily upon our vital energy. Each of us has different demands. In my case I push myself physically because I enjoy activity. I enjoy mental activity. I like challenges. I like problems. I enjoy solving problems. I don't live a soft life physically or mentally. As a man, I am a searcher for spiritual light, for spiritual comforts, tranquillity and serenity. All of this takes energy. Physical activity takes energy of one kind, mental energy takes energy of another kind and spiritual takes energy of yet another kind. So you see one cannot give simple answers when it comes to nutrition. The nutritionist can give a lot of vital information, but the nutritionist cannot eat for you; he cannot digest food for you; he cannot eliminate food for you. What I eat may not suit your likes or dislikes. I don't eat as much food as the average person craves and desires.

Every human being is unique, just as each snowflake falls with matchless design. I am not going to try to persuade you into any one pattern of eating, nevertheless if you want superior health you must eat a diet of superior food. I am not going to tell you to be a raw fooder, a strict vegetarian, a lacto-vegetarian or a mixed eater. As you fast and as you purify your body, the inner-voice, the inner instinct will assert itself. I don't believe that you can jump from a highly refined diet to a natural diet which calls for 50 to 60 percent raw fruits and vegetables. Nature won't heal in sudden jolts. You ate in a certain pattern for many years, your digestive and vital organs have adjusted themselves to this form of food. You have to move along slowly and in time, by body purification through fasting and adhering to the dictates of the 9 Natural Doctors, you will be the same as I am and hundreds of other people that I know...and you will be led instinctively to the selection of natural foods.

You can't eat a nice, fresh combination salad one day and the next day have a big dish of starchy spaghetti. You can't eat a fruit salad one day and load up on hot-dogs and doughnuts the next day. Your nutrition has to be consistent. Let me illustrate what I mean. If you eat meat, I don't think you should eat it over 3 times a week. If you eat eggs, I don't think you should eat over 4 a week. If you drink milk, I think you should gradually eliminate it from your diet, as well as all other dairy products, because man is the only creature that clings to milk after he is weaned.

WORK TOWARDS A BALANCED, NATURAL DIET

Building a good nutritional program is like climbing a ladder, there is the first rung - and that is the elimination of all devitalized, commercial, dead food of civilization - it means the elimination of coffee, tea, alcohol and soft drinks. It means eliminating the amount of animal products you eat daily, the amount of eggs and dairy products. It means adding more raw fruits and vegetables to your diet until the total amount of raw foods is 50 to 60 percent of your diet. As I have stated, in adding more fruits and vegetables to the diet, you have to move with great caution.

This period of discarding the devitalized foods of civilization, and the adding of more raw fruits and vegetables and more properly cooked fruits and vegetables to the diet is known as the "transition period". Most people from childhood until death, live on a diet that is preponderantly on the acid side. The acid produces autointoxication and in turn this toxic material causes aches, pains and degeneration of the body. So, if you have been living on a diet with a lot of cooked foods, such as meats, proteins, eggs, breads, spaghetti, crackers and cookies, again let me warn you not to add too many raw fruits and vegetables to your diet. After each weekly fast, you will find that you will be able to enjoy and be satisfied with more raw fruit and raw vegetables in your diet; because as you fast you will purify.

After 3 months of faithful weekly fasting, you will be able to add at least 40 percent more raw fruits and vegetables to your diet. Remember the raw fruits and vegetables are the purifiers, t cleansers, the detoxifiers. These are the foods that are in a high rate of solar radiation. They dig down into the old pockets of toxic poison and flush them out and that is exactly what we want to do to attain a Superior State of Radiant Health. So you see that diet is not static, diet is constantly changing if you are dieting for internal purification.

People often ask me at my lectures, or write me and say, "Give me the perfect diet". This I cannot do. Eating is of such a personal nature. There are so many likes and dislikes that I can only counsel an individual, if I know what his eating background has been for the last 5 years. I can only suggest that you study the menus that I have submitted with the foods that I have suggested.

Nutrition is like a chain in which all of the essential items are the separate links. If the chain is weak or is broken at any point the whole chain fails. If there are 40 items that are essential in the diet, and one of these is missing, nutrition fails just as truly as it would if half the links were missing. The absolute lack of any item (or of several items) results in ill health and eventually in death. An insufficient amount of any one item is enough to bring distress to the cells and tissues which are most vulnerable to this particular lack. It is not necessary that every item be furnished in required amounts at every meal, or every day, because our bodies always carry some reserves. As soon as the reserves are lost, however, be they large or small, they must be replenished.

I am herewith submitting to you the foods from which you can select to build your daily diet. You can divide your nutrition into one, two or three meals. As I have told you in this treatise, I do not eat breakfast, or if you call a bowl of fresh fruit a breakfast, then my breakfast is fresh fruit. I am not advising this to everyone; some people enjoy a large breakfast and a small lunch. Everyone's nutritional desires are different, but I feel that we do not need breakfast and I have explained it quite fully.

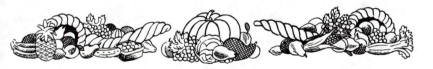

FRUIT - MOST HEALTHFUL FOOD TO MAN

I will start with the fresh fruit list first as I regard fruit as the prize food of man. Fresh fruit or dried fruit can be used as a meal in itself, or it can be used as a dessert with other foods.

FRUIT - PRIZE FOOD OF MAN

Apples (6 varieties)

Apricots (fresh & dried unsulphured)

Avocados

Bananas

Blueberries

Cantaloupes

Casabas

Cherries

Cranberries

Crenshaw Melon

Figs (5 varieties, fresh & dried unsulphured)

Grapefruit (3 varieties)

Grapes (7 varieties)

Honeydew Melon

Kumquats

Lemons & Limes (4 varieties)

Mangos

Nectarines (2 varieties)

Oranges (3 varieties)

Papayas

Peaches (6 varieties fresh & dried) dried)

Pears (6 varieties fresh & dried)

Pineapples (fresh)

Persimmons

Plums (3 varieties fresh & dried)

Prunes (3 varieties fresh & dried)

Raspberries

Strawberries (4 varieties)

Tomatoes (3 varieties)

Watermelon

VEGETABLES - PURIFIERS AND PROTECTORS

In planning perfect health meals, you select the raw vegetables for your salad from this list. For the largest meal of the day, you should select one green and one yellow vegetable or you can select any other 2 vegetables from this list for your cooked vegetables:

Alfalfa Sprouts

Artichokes

Jerusalem Artichokes

Asparagus

Beets

Yellow Wax Beans

Bean Sprouts

Cabbages (5 varieties)

Carrots

Cauliflower

Celery

Chives

Corn

Cucumbers

Dandelion Greens

Egg Plant

Endive

Escarole

Garlic

Green Peas

Kale

Kohl Rabi

Leeks

Lettuce (6 varieties)

Mustard Greens

Okra

Onions

Oyster Plant

Parsnips

Potatoes (3 varieties)

Potatoes (sweet)

Green Peppers

Radishes (3 varieties)

Shallot

Spinach

String Beans

Squash (Many varieties)

Swiss Chard

Tomatoes (3 Varieties)

Turnips

Turnip Greens

Wheat Grass

Watercress

Yams

NUT AND SEED LIST

Nuts and seeds are rich in protein. You can select any 2 of the nuts and seeds when you are planning a meal. If you eat meat you still should not eat it over 3 times weekly, and on the other days you should eat the nuts or seeds as your protein. If you have tender guns and unreliable dentures, then you should purchase a small nut and seed grinding machine to make it easier to masticate, assimilate and digest nuts and seeds.

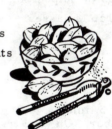

Almonds

Brazil Nuts

Cashew Nuts

Chestnuts

Coconut

Filberts

Hazel Nuts

Peanuts (Roasted if desired)

Pecans

Pinones

Walnuts

Note: All in this group to be purchased and eaten directly from shell, raw and unsalted.

LEGUMES

The legumes are one of man's oldest foods and can be used several times a week as they are rich in vegetable proteins particularly the Soya Bean.

Beans (9 Varieties)

Garbanza Beans

Lentils

Lima Beans

Dried Peas

Split Peas

Soya Beans

★ ★ ★ ★ ★

Perfect health is above gold, and a sound body before riches. —Solomon

OILS

The oils that I have presented in this list are unsaturated and can be used in the diet. Though be sure to read all labels and refuse any oils that contain chemicals to prevent it from going rancid.

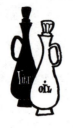

Corn Oil

Peanut Oil

Sesame Seed Oil

Safflower Oil

Soya Oil

Sunflower Oil

Walnut Oil

NATURAL SWEETENING AGENTS

Because I have listed these natural sweetening agents, I want you to remember that they are highly concentrated foods and should be used with great caution.

Clean raw sugar

Yellow D Sugar

Date sugar

Honey

Maple syrup

Molasses (unsulphured)

Blackstrap Molasses

NATURAL WHOLE GRAIN CERALS

Cereals should be used not more than 3 times a week unless you do very heavy physical out-of-door labor. On your whole grain cereal you can use any of the natural sweetening agents.

Barley

Brown Rice

Buckwheat

Corn Meal (yellow & white)

Wheat, Whole, unbleached, unprocessed

Millet

Rye

Flax

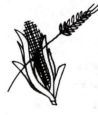

★ ★ ★ ★ ★

In health there is liberty. Health is the first of all liberties, happiness gives us the energy which is the basis of health. — Miel

Corn Bread

Mexican Tortillas (made only from corn)

Millet

100% Rye Bread

100% Whole Wheat Bread

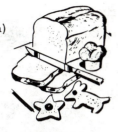

BREADS

I believe that whole grain breads of all kinds should be used with caution, particularly bread made with whole-wheat, because some people cannot tolerate bread, even though it is made of whole grains. People who want to reduce should discontinue all breads, or if they eat bread, the bread should be toasted very dry so the raw starch of the bread is converted into what is known as a grape or blood sugar. People who do sedentary work should limit the amount of bread and toast they use. The only people who seem to be able to tolerate and use more bread than others are those who do very heavy physical labor, particularly those who labor out-of-doors. Limit bread to 2 slices per day.

GUIDE TO EATING MEAT

There are more than 70 varieties of fresh meat from pork, lamb, sheep, calf and beef. From the preponderance of evidence, Nutritionists are agreed that meat is the No. 1 food product. While meat contains protein, it also contains a large amount of cholesterol, which means that cholesterol may find its way into the arteries of the human body and may cause a blockage. Below is a list of the amount of cholesterol per milligrams per 100 grams (3-1/2 ounces).

Brains	2,000	Calves Liver	300
Duck	760	Beef	110
Beef liver	600	Veal	80
Pork-Spareribs	600	Breast of Chicken	80
Kidney	400	Breast of Turkey	80

The person who wants to keep the cholesterol, or blood fat level down, should avoid all meats with thick or fine veins of fat, and remember that even when well-trimmed, "marbled meats" still have a high fat content. Instruct your butcher to closely trim off all visible fats. It is best to do all your own grinding of lean meat. But be sure to avoid meat in which the fat is inextricably bound such as tongue, bacon, rib cuts and others. Today all meat selections must be made by the eye in order to be sure that it is fat free.

DON'T USE		DO USE

DON'T USE

All Fatty Cuts

All Rib Cuts

Tongue: invisible fat

Duck: high both in fat and cholesterol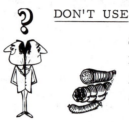

DO USE

All Lean Cuts

Such as:

Lamb - lean

Veal - lean

Beef - Red only

Use organ meat in strict moderation.   Consult cholesterol chart.

 ## DON'T USE

Corned beef

Sausage

Liverwurst

Bologna

Frankfurters

Salami

Pastrami

Luncheon meats

Canned meats

These delicatessen meats are not only high in saturated fats, they are high in salt, used in pickling and preserving, and have a high content of toxic chemicals to prevent decomposition.

If you include meat in your diet do not eat it over 3 times a week. The other times use as your protein the unsaturated natural proteins as found in all nuts and nut meal and nut butters, seeds, such as sunflower, sesame and pumpkin seeds.   Remember that practically all commercial meat is heavily saturated with stilbestrol in order to add additional weight to the animal.   This is a toxic drug.   Meat also carries a high amount of uric acid which is a toxic poison and must be handled by the body.   Meat contains all of the toxic poison that the animal had at the time of slaughter.

FISH LIST

There are about 25 varieties of fish available.   Fish is high in polyunsaturated fats and low in cholesterol.   It is an excellent food which should be served 2 or 3 times a week, if a person selects fish as one of their proteins.   Don't use salted fish such as herring.   In fact don't use any type of salted or dried fish, because of the relatively high cholesterol and salt content.   A very moderate amount of shell fish should be used.   The following list of shell fish contains: milligrams per 100 grams (3-1/2 ounces)

Oyster	325		Shrimp	150	
Lobster	200		Crab	150	

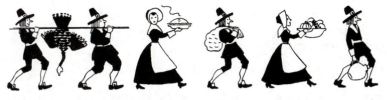

POULTRY LIST

There are about 6 varieties of poultry available on the American market. Chicken and turkey is the best to eat because the fat is less saturated than in lamb and beef fat, and it also contains a fair amount of polyunsaturated fats. Duck and goose is especially high in saturated fat and cholesterol and should be completely avoided by people who want to keep their cholesterol at normal levels.

 ## BEVERAGES

There has always been a controversy whether to drink or not to drink with meals. Personally I think we should do all our drinking between meals and not water-soak our foods. I drink my fruit juices, distilled water and hot herb drinks between meals.

BUILDING A MENU

There are so many different people with so many different desires for food that it is difficult to lay down hard, fast rules for all to follow. As I have explained to you, I eat no breakfast. The only thing I have before noon each day is a bowl of mixed fresh fruits or some kind of stewed fruits such as apricots, prunes, apple-sauce or a baked apple. At lunch I have a raw combination vegetable salad. I will have a dish of cooked greens such as spinach, kale, Swiss Chard, or mustard greens. This is what I call my green vegetable and then I will have a yellow vegetable, such as a yam, sweet potato or yellow squash. With this I will have some sunflower seeds and sesame seeds, or in my grinder, make a meal of these two seeds. For dinner I will have a different type of raw combination vegetable salad. I will have a baked potato and some baked carrots. In other words, I will take my vegetable list and pick out the raw vegetables I am going to use for my raw salad and select any two vegetables to be used for cooking.

With either one of these meals, I can use the raw nut butters, such as blanched almond butter, cashew butter, raw or roasted peanut butter. It has taken many, many years to evolve the diet that I now eat, and I do not want everyone to try and follow my pattern of eating right away - it is a slow process, but so worth the effort.

SAMPLE MENUS

For the person who is used to eating 3 meals a day, I make the following suggestions:

SUGGESTION NO. 1   BREAKFAST

A dish of some kind of fresh fruit, a whole grain cereal, sweetened with either honey or maple syrup; coffee substitute or herb tea sweetened with honey.

LUNCH

A raw vegetable salad; choice of meat, fish or fowl, baked, roasted or broiled. But never fried. One or two cooked vegetables, coffee substitute or herb tea.

     DINNER

Raw vegetable salad, or a fresh fruit salad; choice of meat, fish or fowl, baked, roasted or broiled. Two cooked vegetables, fresh fruit for dessert, coffee substitute or herb tea.

SUGGESTION NO. 2   BREAKFAST

Fresh fruit or unsulphured stewed fruit. One egg, never fried, best method of preparing, hard boiled. Two slices of whole-grain Melba toast, coffee substitute or herb tea.

LUNCH

A raw vegetable salad, baked beef loaf, steamed Zucchini (Italian) squash, cooked string beans, apple-sauce sweetened with honey for dessert. Coffee substitute or herb tea.

DINNER

Raw vegetable salad with diced avocado, tomatoes, cucumbers, lettuce and shredded beets. Lemon, oil or mayonnaise dressing. Green peppers stuffed with brown rice. Choice of any cooked vegetable. Fresh dates for dessert. Coffee substitute or herb tea.

SUGGESTION NO. 3   BREAKFAST

Fresh or stewed fruit, a bran muffin with honey, coffee substitute or herb tea.

     LUNCH

Raw vegetable salad, corn on the cob, baked potato, and a baked apple for dessert. Coffee substitute or herb tea.

DINNER

Raw vegetable or fresh, fruit salad; choice of meat, fish or fowl, baked roasted or broiled. Baked egg plant, mustard greens and stewed tomatoes. Fresh fruit for dessert. Coffee substitute or herb tea.

LARGE VARIETY FOR DELICIOUS - NUTRITIOUS MENUS

It is impossible to take the 200 foods that I have listed, which I feel are good natural foods to eat, and make menus to suit everyone. The thing is to go over the list of foods that you can eat and build your own menus.

People have built up such strong desires for certain foods that it is impossible for them to give up the food that they are most strongly attracted to, of course, I am talking about foods that appear in these lists and not the devitalized foods. The Bible tells us that God provided an ideal diet in the Garden of Eden. It plainly states, "And God said, Behold, I have given you every herb bearing seed which is upon the face of the earth, and every tree, in which is the fruit of a tree yielding seed; to you it shall be for meat".

In other words, God gave man grains, fruits, nuts, seeds and vegetables for a diet that would give health and long-life. We read in the bible that people who lived on this diet lived as many as 900 years. As long as man lived on the simple foods of Nature, he experienced a superior health, a freedom from all ailments, and a long life.

Over the years man started doing things to his natural food. Many of them which he now eats are foodless foods. The further man strayed away from his natural foods, the more trouble he got into. As long as he lived on an abundance of raw fruits and vegetables with properly cooked vegetables, and uncooked, and unprocessed, and unsalted nuts and seeds, he enjoyed a long life and vitality supreme. Natural foods are the only foods that promote the higher health. These are the foods that our digestive system was made for.

The more natural you make your diet, the better health you are going to have. You have 200 foods here to select from, with these foods and your program of fasting, there is no reason why you shouldn't keep in prime physical condition at all times.

★ ★ ★ ★ ★

It (food) probably plays an important part in setting the
pattern of nervous and emotional responses that make
the personality -Human Nutrition, U.S. Dept. of Agriculture

AVOID THESE FOODS

1.   AVOID the use of refined SUGAR.   It provides no nutrients except carbohydrates.   Excessive consumption is a prominent factor in dental decay and reduces the appetite for nourishing food.   Honey may be used with discretion.

2.   AVOID the use of WHITE FLOUR.   It has had the vital elements of the grain removed, and enrichment replaces only a few of them.   Frequently bleaching and preservative agents are added which may be harmful.

3.   AVOID the use of foods such as BREAD, PASTRIES, ICE CREAM, CHEESE, AND COLD MEATS WHICH CONTAIN CHEMICAL ADDITIVES.   These are often used as preservatives, coloring and flavoring agents, emulsifiers, extenders, sweeteners, stabilizers, etc.

4.   AVOID use of POULTRY AND MEATS PRODUCED WITH HORMONES to stimulate growth and add weight.

5.   AVOID the USE OF HYDROGENATED FATS AND OILS. They contain mainly saturated fatty acids.

6.   AVOID HEATED OR PROCESSED MILK, PROCESSED CHEESE, CHEESE FOODS, AND CHOCOLATE.

S U M M A R Y

Today many of our foods are highly processed or refined, thus robbing them of essential vitamins, minerals, and enzymes; some contain harmful chemicals.

The research, findings, and experience of many nutritionists, physicians and dentists have led them to believe that such devitalized foods are a major cause of poor health.   The enormous increase in the last fifty years in degenerative diseases such as heart disease, arthritis, and dental decay, would seem to substantiate this belief.   Scientific research has shown that many of these afflictions may be prevented; and others, when once established, may be arrested or in some cases even reversed through nutritional methods.

★ ★ ★ ★ ★

Simplicity...simplicity...simplicity, let your affairs be as two or three, and not as a hundred or a thousand.

186

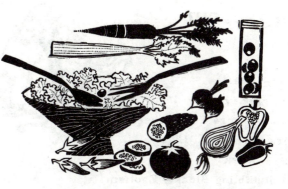

THESE STEPS FOR BETTER HEALTH
THROUGH BETTER FOOD

1. Serve as many foods in the original state as possible - fresh fruits and vegetables, nuts and seeds.

2. PROTEIN

    a. Meat, including the variety meats - liver, kidney, brain, heart - poultry and sea food. Cook meat as little as possible because protein is injured by prolonged high heat.

    b. Dairy products, eggs, unprocessed cheese, and medically Certified raw milk. (Personally I do not use milk or dairy products).

    c. The legumes, soy and other beans.

    d. Nuts and seeds.

3. Use FRUITS and VEGETABLES (grown without the use of poisonous chemical sprays if possible.) Cook vegetables with a minimum of water, at low heat, and for as short a time as possible. Use the liquid.

4. Use freshly ground WHOLEGRAIN CEREALS and FLOURS, for they contain more protein, all of the B complex vitamins, vitamin E, minerals, and unsaturated fatty acids.

5. Use COLD-PROCESSED VEGETABLE OILS, which are an excellent source of essential unsaturated fatty acids.

★ ★ ★ ★ ★

The laws of health are inexorable; we see people going down and out in the prime of life simply because no attention is paid to them. — Paul C. Bragg

FOOD FOR THOUGHT

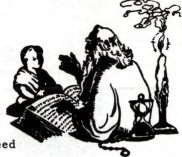

The Great Sin — Fear

The Best Day — Today

The Best Town — Where You Succeed

The Best Work — What You Like

The Best Play — Work

The Greatest Stumbling Block — Egotism

The Greatest Mistake — Giving Up

The Most Expensive Indulgence — Hate

The Greatest Trouble-maker — One Who Talks Too Much

The Most Ridiculous Trait — False Pride

The Most Dangerous Man — The Liar

The Greatest Need — Common Sense

The Greatest Thought — God

The Greatest Wealth — Health

The Greatest Gift You Can Give or Receive — Love

The Greatest Race To Win — A Long Vigorous Life

Man's Greatest Companion and Friend — Good Books

Your Enemies — Envy, Greed, Self-Indulgence, Self-Pity

Life's Greatest Adventure — Growth on the Physical, Mental and Spiritual Plane

Most Disgusting — A Show Off

Most Repulsive — A Bully

Most Overbearing Manner — Arrogance

Man's Greatest Stumbling Block — Ignorance

The Greatest Sieve — Before You Say Anything, Say To Yourself Is It Kind? — Is It True? — Is It Necessary

* THE CLEVEREST MAN *

ONE WHO ALWAYS DOES WHAT HE THINKS IS RIGHT

BE A CLEVER MAN!

"Yet even now," says the Lord, "return to me with all your heart, with fasting..."

--Joel 2:12

31

NATURE KNOWS NO MERCY

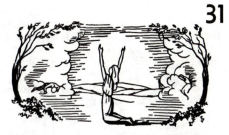

There is no thought or discrimination in the working of the Eternal Laws that govern all things. Evenly, ruthlessly, eternally, Nature works according to fixed laws for good or for ill ... thinking as little of us creatures that build or die on this earth, as the boy at play thinks of the ant hill beneath his foot.

It is for the ant to select a safe, secluded place for her nest, or suffer. It is for us to study Nature's Eternal Laws, and adjust ourselves to them, or suffer. Nature has no time or thought for individual cases. Fire will burn the innocent child and spare the hardened criminal who knows the ways of fire. It is well for us that it is so, for our real education is acquired by the study of the Natural Laws that will not study or spare us.

Unsentimental, regardless of justice or injustice, is powerful Nature in her work on this earth.

She may crush with disease and premature aging the just man and his family who disobeys her laws while sparing the criminal who follows Nature's plan of physical health.

The purpose of this book is to help you save yourself by following the Natural Laws of Living. If we know and follow the Natural Laws that pertain to our life and our health ... we are going to be saved from needless suffering. Although Natural Laws are impersonal, we can cooperate with them and achieve the Highest Health and Live a Long, Vigorous Life!

Nature tells us that we must keep clean inside. That we must not allow toxic poisons, obstructions, water, and morbid poisons to accumulate within our bodies. A regular Fasting Program as given in this book is to teach you the great Law of Internal Purity.

Self Preservation is the first Law of Life. If we are to live a long, healthy, active and happy life ... we must work with Nature and not against her! If you attempt to break her Natural Laws she will break you. Natural Laws are Good

Laws. If we follow them, we will be rewarded with Super Health! Nature demands by strict laws that you keep your bod clean inside and there is no better way to keep the body clean inside than by periodic fasting.

Make Mother Nature your personal friend. Here is a friend that will never, ever fail you if you will work with her and not against her.

If after reading this book it sounds reasonable and intelligent — follow it. Live by it and let no man keep you away from living by these Natural Laws.

WHICH PERSON ARE YOU?

There are only two kinds of people in the world. Which kind are you? The real person thinks for himself. The imitation person lets others think for him?

It takes courage to live your own life. Fasting and Living the Health Life takes courage in this sick, poisoned world. Set a high standard of living for yourself. Demand the best health! Let no weakling drag you down to their level. It is the surviva of the fittest. Be fit, be strong, Live long and vigorously!

Let this book be your guidepost to a Long and Healthy Life. May the knowledge and wisdom in this book bring YOU a New Life; A Life Free From All physical suffering, A Life with Youthful Energy, Peace of Mind, and the Joy of Living.

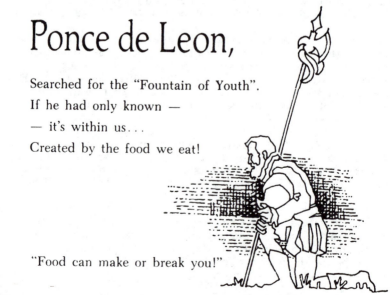

Ponce de Leon,

Searched for the "Fountain of Youth".

If he had only known —

— it's within us...

Created by the food we eat!

"Food can make or break you!"

32

THE SPIRITUAL ASPECTS OF FASTING

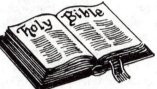

As a crusader on the benefits of fasting for some 70 years, it is indeed gratifying to see the increased interest that has been developing in this subject during the past decade. Not only has the medical profession rediscovered fasting as Nature's primary method of healing, but there is also a reawakening to the important role of fasting in attaining spiritual development.

My own regular program of fasting, as outlined in this book, is one of the basic reasons that I am still here to appreciate this fruition of the Natural Health Crusade . . . alert and ageless in body, mind and spirit as I approach the century mark on the calendar.

During the three-quarters of the 20th century (1900-1975) I have seen human existence become more and more complex . . . technological advances so far outstripping biological adjustment and moral developments that most human beings feel lost and confused. They are groping for stability in the midst of chaos. A sick world is seeking physical, mental and spiritual health.

In time of deep trouble, our natural instincts lead us back to the fundamentals of Natural Law, and usually this return is made with knowledge gained in a hard-learned lesson. Fasting as the means of purifying and healing body, mind and spirit is instinctive with annimals, infants and primitive peoples. Now civilized adult human beings are beginning to learn the power of this simple, natural method. Books and articles are appearing pointing out the spiritual as well as the physical benefits of fasting.

FASTING HEIGHTENS SPIRITUAL AWARENESS

As the body cleanses and heals itself by fasting, keener mental concentration and clearer spiritual perception develop. Remember, the brain is the physical instrument of the mind. When the mucus and toxic poisons are flushed from the brain cells, worries and frustrations are also flushed from your mind. It becomes free and clear. You can think intelligently and logically. Your memory is sharp and keen. Your creative powers are expanded. You are able to face reality and yourself . . . to view your problems objectively and find definite answers — and solutions!

The elimination of toxic wastes releases the mind from physical bondage. The freedom from the necessity of procuring, preparing, eating, digesting and assimilating food releases a tremendous amount of nervous energy which invigorates the mental and spiritual processes. You attain new levels of tranquility, serenity and peace of mind. You become spiritually perceptive and receptive.

You can become at one with the Infinite . . . "Be still, and know that I am God."

"Fasting does not change God, but man. A cleansing process takes place. The awareness of the purification of the heart builds faith, and faith in God means authority with God." So states Rev. Charles F. Stanley, Atlanta, Georgia, in a recent article. (*Fasting*, MOODY MONTHLY, May 1975).

In *God's Chosen Fast* (Christian Literature Crusade, Ft. Washington, Pa.) author Arthur Wallis says:

"Without doubt there is a very close connection between the practice of fasting and the receiving of spiritual revelation. Many non-Christian religions such as Buddhism, Hinduism, Confucianism and Islam (also) practice fasting because they know its power to detach one's mind from the world of sense, and to sharpen one's sensibility to the world of spirit."

GREAT SPIRITUAL LEADERS PRACTICED FASTING

It was after fasting for forty days and forty nights that Moses received the Ten Commandments on Mt. Sinai. Jesus spent forty days and forty nights of fasting in the desert before starting His ministry.

The founders of the world's four religions of today -- Christianity, Judaism, Buddhism and Islam -- taught fasting as a means of communication with the Divine through purification of body, mind and spirit...to be carried out with dedication and in private.

Similar teachings are to be found in nearly all religions, ancient and tribal, as well as influential philosophies and moral codes. Zoroaster, the great Persian prophet, taught and practiced fasting. So did Plato, Socrates and Aristotle. Hippocrates, the father of medicine, considered fasting to be the great natural healer. The genius Leonardo da Vinci practiced and advocated fasting.

China's great philosopher and teacher, Confucius, included fasting in his precepts. The Yogis of India and the American Indians practice fasting as a means of spiritual enlightenment.

The greatest modern example of the power of fasting is Mahatma Ghandi, who won India's freedom from the great British Empire in a complete and non-violent victory of spiritual leadership.

MY UNFORGETTABLE EXPERIENCE WITH GHANDI

The date was July 27, 1946 in New Delhi, which would become the capital of the new Republic of India a year and a month later. (India's independence became official on August 15, 1947.) At Ghandi's headquarters here I received permission to accompany this amazing man on a 21-day fasting trip eastward through the villages, where he would talk with the people and help them with their problems. At that time the average Indian earned about 10 cents a day, and starvation was a way of life. To show he shared their plight, this saintly and compassionate spiritual leader was planning to travel the dusty roads from village to village on foot, without food, for three weeks.

Ghandi was then 77 years of age, and very frail in apperance. But looks were indeed deceiving. This man was a tower of strength . . . physically, mentally and spiritually. His stamina, endurance and energy were astounding.

The trek began at sunup. The heat and humidity were the worst I have ever experienced . . . and I have spent time in some of the hottest spots in the world, including Death Valley in California, the Sahara Desert, and an 800-mile bicycle trip across North Africa in intense summer heat. But never once did Ghandi seem to tire, never once did he falter in his fast pace of walking.

The only time he sat down was during talks with the villagers. He would speak for 20 minutes, then answer questions for another 20 minutes. Then off down the hot, dusty road the Ghandi party would go to the next village. He ate nothing, and drank only water flavored with lemon and honey.

Is this not the fast that I choose: to loose the bonds of wickedness, to undo the thongs of the yoke, to let the oppressed go free and to break every yoke?

--Isaiah 58:6

Many who tried to travel with him fell by the wayside from heat and exhaustion. But Ghandi was inexhaustible. I have been an athlete all my life and a high mountain climber . . . but I have never seen a human who had the physical staying power and limitless energy as Ghandi. He walked and talked until sundown before he stopped for a rest.

In the days that I was a member of the Ghandi party I had many talks with him on the power of fasting. Of the number of things I learned from him this statement seems to me the summation:

"All the vitality and all the energy I have comes to me because my body is purified by fasting."

Walking mile after mile from village to village, he gave the people hope and courage that a better life was coming to them. His internal strength was so powerful that weak people felt strong after seeing him and hearing his words. He gave of his unlimited strength to the discouraged and the sick. He brought bright light where there was darkness.

Ghandi told the people to fast and purify their bodies, and regardless of their circumstances they would find peace and joy on earth.

"Fasting will bring spiritual rebirth to those of you who cleanse and purify your bodies," he told those who thronged to hear him. "The light of the world will illuminate within you when you fast and purify yourself."

This trip with the great Mahatma Ghandi is an experience I will never forget. This physically small man was a spiritual giant. He led the millions of people on the sub-continent of India to independence from the mighty British Empire without striking a single physical blow. And yet, with all his power and influence, he was completely without arrogance. Characteristically, on the day of India's independence, Ghandi took no part in the celebrations that went on throughout the country . . . but spent the day in fasting and prayer.

THE GROTTO WHERE JESUS FASTED

On one of my trips to the Holy Land, I was in the area of Jericho on an archeological research project. It was near the Mount of Temp -tation, the mountaintop where Jesus is said to have been tempted by the devil after his fast of forty days and forty nights, and I determined to climb it. It was a long but easy ascent. From the top, which was still 200 feet below sea level, I looked down upon the terrible, hot, bleached bareness of the Jordan Valley.

He fasted forty days and forty nights, and afterward he was hungry.   *--Matthew 4:2*

On my descent, halfway down the mountain, built partly within the rock itself, I came upon a monastery where ten elderly Greek monks were living in poverty. Following the ancient custom of greeting any stranger as if he might be the wandering Christ, these monks welcomed me with beautiful courtesy. I was taken on a tour of the monastery. It was a fantastic place . . . parts of it jutting out over deep, brutal chasms . . . other rooms carved out of the solid rock.

One of these was a grotto which, the guide told me, was "the very spot where Jesus fasted forty days and forty nights, and was tempted by the devil."

The monks told me that they fasted two days every week, and once a year fasted forty days and nights in the grotto. They felt that this fasting had not only given them great spiritual enlightenment, but had also added many vigorous years to their lives.

Their appearance bore them out. Although far along in calendar years, these men had great flexibility in their bodies. It required a lot of physical stamina to keep the monastery in good condition in this rugged, barren wilderness and oven heat. All were lean and muscular, with the glow of health to their skin and bright, keen eyes —none wore glasses.

Their spiritual quality showed in the genuine brotherly love which they bestowed on me, a stranger. At the end of my visit, one of the monks escorted me to the gate, kissed me on both cheeks, and gave me a blessing in Greek.

Looking back, as I descended the long, stony trail, I saw him watching solicitously. We waved to each other, and I carried a warm glow of friendliness in my heart from that barren rocky land.

Here again was proof of what I have learned from my own experience...that one of the spiritual benefits of fasting is a genuine sense of the kinship of all humanity.

THE FAST OF 40 DAYS AND 40 NIGHTS

There is a significance to the "forty days and forty nights" of fasting of the great spiritual leaders and of those who seek the highest spiritual enlightenment. This is the practical limit to which the disciplined body can exist without food before it begins to consume itself. The cleansing process has been completed . . . toxic wastes and excess fat have been "incinerated", burned up into energy. When this limit is reached, starvation begins . . . the body will have to feed on sound living tissue . . . and this is harmful to body, mind and spirit. The fast should be terminated before this point is reached! _____

I humbled my soul with fasting.   *--Psalm 69:10*

A long fast should not be attempted until the body has been trained to fast for short intervals . . . a day to a week . . . over a considerable period of time. The 40-days-and-nights fast is not for the novice.

The experienced faster learns to distinguish between the early cravings of appetite and the warning pangs of real hunger.

At the beginning of a fast there is a craving for food which arises from the habit of eating at certain intervals. This may last for several days, then the craving passes. There follows a short period of several days or more when the faster feels weak and faint, and requires a great deal of rest. This is probably the most difficult part of the fasting experience.

Gradually this sense of weakness disappears, signalling that the body has eliminated its grosser wastes and poisons. Then comes a feeling of growing strength, with little or no concern about food, and an increasing mental alertness. There is a sense of release and freedom, and one ascends to higher levels of serenity and peace of mind. Spritual awareness can reach a point of ecstasy.

How long this period lasts depends upon the individual. When the process of elimination of all wastes has been completed, the body signals a warning with pangs of genuine hunger. When this happens, whether in two weeks or forty days, the fast must end in order to preserve its benefits!

A SOUND MIND IN A SOUND BODY

Even the greatest spiritual leaders that the world has known trained themselves by habitual fasting of one or two days per week before they undertook longer fasts. Herein lies the difference between genuine fasting and extreme asceticism, which has given fasting a bad name by prolonging it into starvation.

True fasting is psychosomatic . . . *psycho,* mind or spirit; *soma,* body . . . a natural means of achieving "a sound mind in a sound body,"as the Greeks put it. Or, according to the Bible, "Your body is a temple of the Holy Spirit."

To quote again from Dr. Stanley:

"Because the body is the temple of the Holy Spirit, it demands the best of care. According to medical experts, fasting is the most natural, original process of purifying the body. Since the Lord admonished man to work six days and rest one, would it not be equally wise to rest the digestive system for one day as well? I believe so.

"I have found that fasting also sharpens the mind. The physical and spiritual benefits cannot be separated. A clear mind is essential to the desire for oneness and direction."

On a fast day...you shall read the words of the Lord.
--Jeremiah 36:6

And from Arthur Wallis:

"...Our physical condition can often influence our spiritual lives more than we realize....Is God glorified when (our bodies) are weak or sickly through neglect of the divine laws that govern their well-being? Is God glorified when we become 'casualties' in the fight through over-working, over-feeding or undernourishing our bodies, and failing to give them their 'sabbath' of rest and relaxation?

"In an age of pressure, when the breakdown of mind or body . . . is becoming all too familiar, the physical (as well as the spiritual) value of a fast of God's choosing becomes a matter of some importance. Here is a divine provision for health and healing, for renewal of mind and body, that we must further consider."

Courage, vitality, energy, endurance, zest and vigor...these are not mental states to be conjured up at will, but are the mental expression of a physical state. The Bible tells us that the "the kingdom of heaven is within." Fasting purifies all the 40 trillion cells of the body, including those of the brain. When the brain is free from toxic poisons the mind is liberated, psychologically and spiritually. It is free from anxieties, boredom, loneliness, tension and fear. It can meet all of life's problems and make wise decisions. It can find deep contentment . . . realize a fuller, more meaningful, happier life.

Fasting is a natural tranquilizer with absolutely no side effects. A brain purified by fasting pays higher dividends than any other investment you can make. Begin today! Let this book be your guide! Discover the Miracle of Fasting!

★ ★ ★ ★ ★

Our sincere blessings to you dear friends, who make our lives so worthwhile and fulfilled by reading our teachings on natural living as our Creator laid down for us all to follow . . . Yes—he wants us all to follow the simple path of natural living and this is what we teach in our books and health crusades world-wide. Our prayers reach out to you for the best in health and happiness for you and your loved ones. This is the birthright He gives us all . . . but we must follow the laws He has laid down for us, so we can reap this precious health, physically, mentally and spiritually!

Paul C. Bragg   *Patricia Bragg*

★ ★ ★ ★ ★

"Teach me Thy way, O Lord;
and lead me in a plain path . . ."
Psalms 97:11

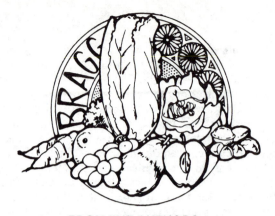

FROM THE AUTHORS

This book was written for YOU. It can be your passport to the Good Life. We Professional Nutritionists join hands in one common objective — a high standard of health for all and many added years to your life. Scientific Nutrition points the way — Nature's Way — the only lasting way to build a body free of degenerative diseases and premature aging. This book teaches you how to work with Nature and not against her. Doctors, dentists, and others who care for the sick, try to repair depleted tissues which too often mend poorly if at all. Many of them praise the spreading of this new scientific message of natural foods and methods for long-lasting health and youthfulness at any age. To speed the spreading of this tremendous message, this book was written.

Statements in this book are recitals of scientific findings, known facts of physiology, biological therapeutics, and reference to ancient writings as they are found. Paul C. Bragg has been practicing the natural methods of living for over 70 years, with highly beneficial results, knowing they are safe and of great value to others, and his daughter Patricia Bragg works with him to carry on the Health Crusade. They make no claims as to what the methods cited in this book will do for one in any given situation, and assume no obligation because of opinions expressed.

No cure for disease is offered in this book. No foods or diets are offered for the treatment or cure of any specific ailment. Nor is it intended as, or to be used as, literature for any food product. Paul C. Bragg and Patricia Bragg express their opinions solely as Public Health Educators, Professional Nutritionists and Teachers.

Certain persons considered experts may disagree with one or more statements in this book, as the same relate to various nutritional recommendations. However, any such statements are considered, nevertheless, to be factual, as based upon long-time experience of Paul C. Bragg and Patricia Bragg in the field of human health.

From time to time, the Braggs send out startling New Discoveries in the field of Nutrition, Health and Physical Fitness. Send your name, address and zip code for these Free announcements to:

HEALTH SCIENCE, Box 7, Santa Barbara, California 93102 U.S.A.

SEND FOR IMPORTANT
FREE HEALTH BULLETINS

Patricia Bragg, from time to time sends News Bulletins on latest Health and Nutrition Discoveries. These are sent *free of charge!*

If you wish to receive these *free bulletins* and The Health Builder— please send your name and also names of any friends and relatives you wish.

HEALTH SCIENCE Box 7, Santa Barbara, California 93102 U.S.A.

Name

Address

City   State   Zip Code

Name

Address

City   State   Zip Code

Name

Address

City   State   Zip Code

Name

Address

City   State   Zip Code

Name

Address

City   State   Zip Code

PLEASE CUT ALONG DOTTED LINE

Bragg

Live Longer — Healthier — Stronger
Self - Improvement Library

Let Legendary PAUL C. BRAGG, World Health Crusader, Pioneer Nutritionist, Originator of Health Stores and Beloved Sage to Millions and PATRICIA BRAGG, Health and Fitness Educator, Show You the Simple Path to a Greater, Longer, More Vital Life — "High Health" Physically, Mentally and Spiritually!

BRAGG "HOW-TO, SELF-HEALTH" BOOKS

__ Vegetarian Gourmet Health Recipes (Delicious Hi-Protein, no salt, no sugar) . . . $4.95

__ Bragg's Complete Health Gourmet Recipes - 448 pages 6.95

__ The Miracle of Fasting (Bragg Bible of Health) 4.95

__ Complete Triathlon Endurance Training Manual - 600 pages . . . . Hard Cover 24.95

    (This Bragg Health/Fitness Encyclopedia is a must reading for all!) . . Soft Cover 16.95

__ Building Powerful Nerve Force 4.95

__ How to Keep the Heart Healthy and Fit at Any Age 4.95

__ The Golden Keys to Internal Physical Fitness 2.95

__ The Natural Way to Reduce 4.95

__ The Shocking Truth About Water 4.95

__ Your Health and Your Hair 4.95

__ Healthful Eating Without Confusion 4.95

__ Salt-Free Sauerkraut Recipes 2.95

__ Nature's Healing System to Improve Eyesight in 90 days 4.95

__ Building Strong Feet 2.95

__ Super Brain Breathing for Vital Living 1.75

__ Toxicless Diet — Body Purification & Healing System (Stay Ageless Program) 2.95

__ Powerful Health Uses of Apple Cider Vinegar 2.95

__ Building Health & Youthfulness 1.75

__ Natural Method of Physical Culture 1.75

__ Nature's Way to Health — Live 100 Active Years 1.75

__ Fitness Program with Spine Motion — for Flexible, Youthful, Painfree Back 1.95

__ The New Science of Health for Peace of Mind 1.75

__ The Philosophy of Super Health 1.75

__ South Sea Culture of the Abdomen for Perfect Elimination & Trim Waist 1.75

Prices subject to change without notice

Remember . . . The Gift of a Bragg Book is a Gift of Life!

Buy these Bragg books today for yourself, family and friends. Purchase or order at your health store or better book stores. If unavailable in your area, you may obtain from Health Science. When ordering please add for postage and handling — $1.00 for first, 50¢ for each additional book. Remittance in U.S. funds only. California residents add sales tax.

HEALTH SCIENCE
Box 7, Santa Barbara, California 93102 U.S.A.

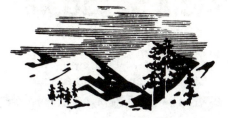

TEN HEALTH COMMANDMENTS

Thou shall respect thy body as the highest manifestation of Life.

Thou shall abstain from all unnatural, devitalized food and stimulating beverages.

Thou shall nourish thy body with only Natural, unprocessed, "live" food, — that . . .

Thou shall extend thy years in health for loving, charitable service.

Thou shall regenerate thy body by the right balance of activity and rest.

Thou shall purify thy cells, tissue and blood with pure fresh air and sunshine.

Thou shall abstain from ALL food when out of sorts in mind or body.

Thou shall keep thy thoughts, words and emotions, pure, calm and uplifting.

Thou shall increase thy knowledge of Nature's laws, abide therewith, and enjoy the fruits of thy life's labor.

Thou shall lift up thyself and thy brother man with thine own obedience to God's Natural, Pure Laws of Living.

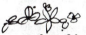

Our sincere blessings to you dear friends, who make our lives so worthwhile and fulfilled by reading our teachings on natural living as our Creator laid down for us all to follow . . . Yes—he wants us all to follow the simple path of natural living and this is what we teach in our books and health crusades world-wide. Our prayers reach out to you for the best in health and happiness for you and your loved ones. This is the birthright He gives us all . . . but we must follow the laws He has laid down for us, so we can reap this precious health, physically, mentally and spiritually!

Paul C. Bragg   *Patricia Bragg*

Open thou mine eyes, that I may behold wondrous things out of thy law.—Psalm 119:18

PATRICIA BRAGG, N.D., Ph.D.

Lecturer and Author
Nutritionist, Educator, Health & Fitness Consultant
Advisor to World Leaders, Glamorous Hollywood Stars,
Singers, Dancers and Athletes

Daughter of the world renowned health authority, Paul C. Bragg, Patricia Bragg has won international fame on her own in this field. She conducts Health and Fitness Seminars for women's, men's, youth and church groups throughout the United States ... and is co-lecturer with Paul C. Bragg on tours throughout the English speaking world. Consultants to Presidents and Royalty, to Stars of Stage, Screen and TV, and to Champion Athletes, Patricia Bragg and her father are authors and co-authors of the Bragg Health Library of instructive, inspiring books.

Patricia Bragg herself is the symbol of perpetual youth, a living and sparkling example of hers and her father's precepts.

A fifth generation Californian on her mother's side, Patricia Bragg was reared by the Natural Health Method from infancy. In school, she not only excelled in athletics but also won high honors in her studies and her counseling. She is an accomplished musician and dancer ... as well as tennis player, swimmer and mountain climber ... and the youngest woman ever to be granted a U.S. Patent. Patricia Bragg is a popular gifted Health Teacher and a dynamic, in-demand Talk Show Guest. In the past few years she has been featured on over 300 radio talk shows spreading simple easy-to-follow health teachings for everyone. Man's body is the Temple of the Holy Spirit, and our Creator wants us filled with Joy and Health for a long walk with him for Eternity. The Bragg Crusade of Health and Fitness (3 John 2) has carried her around the world ... spreading health and joy physically, spiritually and mentally. Health is our birthright, and Patricia teaches how to prevent the destruction of our health from man-made wrong habits of living.

She has been Health Consultant to that great walker, President Harry S. Truman, and to the British Royal Family. Betty Cuthbert, Australia's "Golden Girl" who holds 16 world records and four Olympic gold medals in women's track, follows Patricia Bragg's guidance. Among those who come to her for advice are some of Hollywood's top stars from Clint Eastwood and family to the singing stars of the Metropolitan Opera. Patricia's message is of world-wide appeal to people of all ages, nationalities and walks-of-life who read her books and attend her Crusades.

Jesus said: "Thy faith hath made thee whole, and go and sin no more." And that means your dietetic sins. He himself, through fasting and prayer, was able to heal the sick and cure all manner of diseases.

Dear friend, I wish above all things that thou may prosper and be in health even as the soul prosper—
3 John 2